The Bonding through Pregnancy

How to make your mate, feel absolutely great!

This is a book by Cruze Weston.

www.cruzeweston.com

If you like this book,

Then chances are that you'll like my other books too. I created a private book club where members get early releases for free; for an exchange of their thoughts and ideas.

You can become a member of the Cruze Weston Club and start getting free books by visiting www.cruzeweston.com/club

Table of Contents

It's Really Happening	7
Chapter 1: Those Two Little Words	10
The first month:	10
What's up with your partner:	12
What's up with the peanut:	16
What's up with you:	17
Key things to do this month:	18
Nice things to do for your partner this month:	23
Easy dad recipes to make:	25
Chapter 2: Rolling Right Along	27
The second month:	27
What's up with your partner:	28
What's up with the peanut:	31
What's up with you:	32
Key things to do this month:	33
Nice things to do for your partner this month:	35
Easy dad recipes to make:	36
Chapter 3: Finishing Up the First Trimester	39

The third month:	39
What's up with your partner:	42
What's up with the peanut:	43
What's up with you:	44
Key things to do this month:	44
Nice things to do for your partner this month:	46
Easy dad recipes to make:	48
Chapter 4: The Second Trimester	49
The fourth month:	49
What's up with your partner	50
What's up with the peanut:	51
What's up with you:	52
Key things to do this month:	53
Nice things to do for your partner this month:	55
Easy dad recipes to make:	56
Chapter 5: The Halfway Mark	59
The fifth month:	59
What's up with your partner:	59
What's up with the peanut	61
What's up with you:	62

Key things to do this month:	63
Nice things to do for your partner this month:	65
Easy dad recipes to make:	67
Chapter 6: Growing Baby, Growing Belly	69
The sixth month:	69
What's up with your partner:	70
What's up with the peanut:	71
What's up with you:	72
Key things to do this month:	73
Nice things to do for your partner this month:	74
Easy dad recipes to make:	75
Chapter 7: The Third Trimester	77
The seventh month:	77
What's up with your partner:	77
What's up with the peanut:	79
What's up with you:	80
Key things to do this month	81
Nice things to do for your partner this month:	82
Easy dad recipes to make:	83
Chapter 8: Home Stretch	86

The eighth month:	86
What's up with your partner	86
What's up with the peanut:	89
What's up with you:	90
Key things to do this month:	91
Nice things to do for your partner this month:	92
Easy dad recipes to make:	93
Chapter 9: Here Comes Baby	96
The ninth month:	96
What's up with your partner:	98
What's up with the peanut:	99
What's up with you:	100
Key things to do this month:	101
Nice things to do for your partner this month:	102
Easy dad recipes to make:	103
The Baby is Finally Here!	105
What's up with your partner:	105
What's up with the peanut:	107
What's up with you:	110
Key things to do now:	111

Nice things to do for your partner:	112
Easy dad recipes to make:	113
Helpful Tips and Information	114
Hospital Bag Checklist:	115
Items to Include in a Birth Plan:	117
Great Foods During Pregnancy	119
Realistic Dad Information:	121

It's Really Happening

When it comes to being pregnant, let's face it, men will never know 99% of how it feels. We can watch, we can feel the baby kick, we can hold her hand when she's screaming about how horrible we are as she goes through labor, and we can eat weird things right along with her. In fact, most men don't really know what to do or how to help when their partner is pregnant. I sure didn't that first time around.

Our first pregnancy was a breeze. Seriously. Everything went exactly by the book, my wife wasn't too sick, and labor was pretty easy on her. I thought that just doing a little more to help and cooking dinner – i.e. ordering pizza – was all I had to do. My wife still did everything she normally did, even went to work up to a week before the due date. We thought that every pregnancy was like this and couldn't wait to have another kiddo once our first one was a little bit older. Once he hit two and a half, my wife hit me with the news that she was pregnant for the second time. We were both elated! Surely everything would be as easy as the first one.

Wrong.

The second time around was a complete 180 from the first. It was the extreme opposite of her first pregnancy. She was so sick the entire time, put on bed rest halfway through, and so many other issues that made it hard to enjoy this time around. I had to read, and reread, everything I could find about hard pregnancies and still didn't know anything that I could do to help. To make matters worse, pizza was on the no-no list of things she couldn't even stand to smell. Plus, having her home in bed made me worry more when I was gone, and I ended up with an ulcer at 27 – and I don't recommend the ulcer. Her due date came and went, and her OBGYN finally decided to induce her – which I don't recommend either. The medications they gave my wife to start labor were horrible on her and she ended up in labor for over 36 hours. Our second son was perfect however, and that seemed to make up for everything once we saw that tiny screaming face.

We both decided after that pregnancy, we were done. No more kids. We now had two perfect little boys and we were happy. In fact, we'd forgotten just how bad that second pregnancy was on my wife.

Until we found out she was pregnant for the third time.

I'm not going to lie, I was nervous, scared, excited, and anxious all at the same time. I walked around worried for my wife, feeling like I wanted to puke and jump for joy. I really thought that this one would be as bad as that second time around.

Again, I was wrong.

It amazed me just how different each of these three pregnancies were. The third one measured in between the first and the second, with everything being a bit easier, but not quite as easy as that first kiddo. I will tell you that the labor aspect of the third one went faster than we really planned, we barely made it to the hospital and our daughter was born just a little under an hour later.

My point with this introduction is this: learn everything you can, even if you don't think it will ever happen to you. While I read a lot during that second pregnancy, there just wasn't much out there to help guys know what do to. After our third child, I decided to write this short guide that would help put you on the right path as far as what expectant dads can and should do. You'll find that this book contains as much information on how to help your partner as it does facts about pregnancy. I did learn a lot of these things the hard way and I don't want anyone else to try and guess what they should do.

Armed with these tips, tricks, and information here in this book, you will easily be able to help your partner during her pregnancy and ensure that you're doing all you can to make her comfortable.

Good luck!

Chapter 1: Those Two Little Words

The first month:

She just hit you with those two words: I'm pregnant. Right now, you nervous and over the moon all at once. You're also overwhelmed and wondering what the hell you do next. Let me start by saying this: you need to know up front that pregnancy isn't fun. If you take a deep look at what women go through as opposed to what we go through, there's not even a contest as to who has it easier. She goes through all the bodily changes, the mood swings, the sleepless nights, the cravings, the sickness, the always-have-to-pee stops, the baby kicking her in the ribs, has to go through some of the worst pain ever in labor, or have major surgery to have the baby, and so much more.

Start looking at the timeline of your next nine months now. If you don't already have a calendar where you can physically see dates and write in appointments, get one now. You have no idea how valuable this will be as things get more hectic and you start confusing dates and times – and you will, trust me.

Now is also the time to start looking at the time line of the pregnancy. Chances are that she has a pretty good idea of when she got pregnant, if not, don't worry. At the first doctor visit, they can pinpoint a better date for you and calculate her due date. For now, let's break things down into trimesters, months, and weeks:

Trimester One = Months One, Two and Three = Weeks 1 to 13
Trimester Two = Months Four, Five and Six = Weeks 14 to 26
Trimester Three = Months Seven, Eight and Nine = Weeks 27 to 36-40

Broken down into a simple table makes it seem like a long time. Nine month or up to 40 weeks. However, this time will fly by and you don't want to be looking at the hospital room thinking that you still have so much to do. (You will probably think that anyway, but you can be as prepared as possible.)

What's up with your partner:

She just found out something exciting and life changing as well – and has no idea what to feel aside from that. The first month is more spent trying to make sure that she really is pregnant by doctor's visits and pregnancy tests. In fact, she may go through several at home tests before she ever makes an appointment. No matter how many times she asks for you to go buy one, do it.

Most women won't even know they are pregnant until they miss that first period. So, she could already be a few weeks pregnant before either of you even realize it. She may have no symptoms at all and seem full of energy instead.

However, there are some symptoms that appear pretty soon after she becomes pregnant, even before a period is missed. Here are some of the most common pregnancy signs:

- Sore breasts: This can be anywhere from mild to excruciating. Some women chalk this sign up to PMS, but it's an extremely common symptom of pregnancy. If she mentions the girls are sore, be extra careful when you're around them.
- Darkening areolas: Along with tenderness, the areolas (areas around the nipple) begin to grow larger and darken. Her body will do all sorts of

changing to get ready for the baby. This change is to accommodate breast feeding.
- Fatigue: Is she extremely tired yet you guys haven't done any hiking, running, moving, or other strenuous exercises? Fatigue is one of the key symptoms of pregnancy and she may sleep a lot during the next nine months.
- Bloating: Sure, you both get too full on spaghetti night, but who doesn't? Well, if she is feeling bloated constantly and it's not close to her period, this is an easy sign of pregnancy.
- Increased gas: Yes, it's just a fact of being pregnant and this symptom begins almost immediately as well since her body is already changing to accommodate a munchkin on board.
- Heartburn: Right along the digestive line, heartburn is one of the most common, and painful, symptoms of being pregnant. It will stick around throughout the whole nine months and probably beyond. At the first sign of it, I recommend stocking up on antacids and keeping them throughout the house.
- Cramping: This may be dismissed as normal menstrual cramps at first, but if they continue or if no period comes, it's a pretty good sign that she is pregnant.
- Urinary problems or constipation: Another wonderful sign of pregnancy is more issues

with the digestive tract.
- Nausea: As I mentioned before, some women will have morning sickness hit them right away before they even realize they are pregnant. Usually nausea will hit first thing in the morning, but it can last throughout the day. If it is extremely bad, her doctor can prescribe some medication to help. (They even have a prescription nausea medicine that you rub on your wrists instead of swallowing.)
- Sensitive to smells: While this goes along with nausea, it also is a whole new symptom on its own. She may notice that smells overwhelm her now when she never really noticed them before. This can be good or bad – as good smells can make her happier while bad smells, well, read the bullet point before this one.
- Headaches: Headaches and migraines are things that increase during pregnancy and can become extremely hard on her. Make sure that you're offering to help as much as possible if she has one.
- Dizziness: Many women experience dizzy spells when they are first pregnant. Make sure that she takes it easy if she has a dizzy spell because falling isn't a good thing at any point in a pregnancy.

Keep in mind that she is going through some emotional changes, such as mood swings, as well as physical ones. Some women will begin to have morning sickness while others won't see much change at all. If any of these symptoms develop into a problem that is affecting her daily life, such as work, or other areas, speak to her doctor right away so she can get some relief. Her doctor will also have great information on what she should do to help specific symptoms beyond just medications.

If she is taking any prescription medications, have her call her doctor and find out which ones she should and should not take while pregnant. Chances are that if there is one that's on the no-no list, her doctor can easily find another to take its place. This also includes some products that contain vitamin A, Retin-A, and a few others. If you or she have a question about something, ask her doctor.

She should also consider getting a flu shot if it's getting close to that time of year. You want to have everyone in your immediate family get a flu shot if they will be around her during the pregnancy. Having the flu while pregnant is not only beyond miserable, it can cause complications if it gets too bad.

What's up with the peanut:

While just getting started, that tiny egg is beginning to form a blastocyst, which is a large ball of cells. This ball will already contain the DNA it needs to create your beautiful new kiddo. The DNA contained inside already have determined the sex, eye color, hair and many other traits from both parents. As the month continues, it will begin to form into an embryo and be about the size of a poppy seed. This group of around one hundred cells will begin to grow crazy fast. The inner layer of the cells will become the embryo and the outer layer will become the placenta. At about three weeks, the blastocyst, or baby ball, will begin to burrow into a specific spot where it can grow and have nutrients from its mom.

By the end of the first month, a face is already starting to form, with large dark circles where the eyes will be, the mouth, jaw, and throat are beginning to shape, and even blood cells and circulation will start. Your little peanut will be safely inside the amniotic sac, which gradually fills with fluid and acts as a cushion for the baby. If you were able to see it at this point, your baby would be about the size of a grain of rice.

What's Up With You:

Of course, this doesn't mean that you just sit on the couch and ignore everything. You're going to be stressed out, elated, emotional, scared, bragging to everyone, anxious, and every other feeling that you can think of, during the next nine months. Don't feel bad for going through these emotions. They're normal. Every partner goes through them when their significant other is pregnant. It's just part of it.

However, here is one thing that I learned the hard way: don't vent any negative feelings or thoughts to your pregnant partner. She is already worrying more than you can imagine and dealing with bodily changes on top of that. Keep your comments loving, helpful, and supportive. If you do need to vent, talk to a friend or family member. There's no need to stress her out further.

During the first month, you're mainly getting used to the idea that you're going to be a dad. Everyone who already knows will be ecstatic and congratulating you over and over again. Don't be put out if people are doting on her more than you though. Just remember that she will be the center of attention and will have the most to deal with. Don't fret about it. If you feel like you aren't being as involved as you want to be, make sure that you talk with her about what more you can do to help out, how you can be involved in planning certain things, and so on. Just make sure that you talk about it in a positive way.

Key things to do this month:

Be Supportive: The key thing to remember now and throughout the pregnancy is to be supportive. Do everything that you can to help her be comfortable and know that you're there. Take time to give her a foot rub, bring her something to drink when she needs it, offer to go pick up items she needs at the store. Anything that you can do to make things easier on her will help you both. She is going to be increasingly uncomfortable and just plain miserable at times as the pregnancy progresses.

Go to doctor's appointments: There are going to be more doctor's appointments than you can imagine right now and you need to try to be at every single one. I understand that you can't always get off work, but try to make all that you can. If you can't be there, make sure that she has someone go with her to help remember everything the doctor says. It's helpful to have an extra set of ears as there is so much information in each appointment.

These appointments will include regular checkups for her, visits that monitor the baby's progress, ultrasounds, blood work, other testing, visiting the hospital, and so on. You want to be as prepared as possible, so knowing everything the doctor says is key.

Keep a notebook: I highly recommend keeping a notebook with you constantly. There will always be questions that pop up that you both want to ask the doctor on the next visit. There will also be things that you need to remember to do. Plus, that notebook will be a huge help when you're at the doctor, as you can also jot down the information so you can research it later.

In the back of the notebook, you also should start keeping a list of names that both of you come up with along the way. Of course, this will change every day sometimes, but it's helpful to have a list of what you've already thought of when it's time to make that big decision.

Daydream with your partner: What? Yes, you read that right. Take time just talking about what you think the baby will look like, will it be a boy or a girl, what do you both envision the nursery to look like, and so on. Just this fun relaxing talk can help both of you calm nerves and bond. Make sure that you steer clear of topics like 'what all can go wrong with the labor'. If that comes up, say something like "Let's not worry about that right now" and move on to another happy subject.

Routine changes: It doesn't matter how long you two

have been together, you know that you both have routines that you do throughout your time at home during the day. Take note of where you can jump in and help. There will be things that become harder and harder for her to do as the pregnancy moves on. Dr. Paul Woods, MD told WebMD "Expect that things she used to do are no longer easy for her to do; and even if she's willing, she won't be able to do as much." Dr. Woods is a father of four and understands how these things go. He also says, "You'll willingly need to step up to the plate and do more things around the house than ever before." Yes, this will mean routine changes for you both, and occasionally you both should keep in mind that you can leave a few things until tomorrow if you're both exhausted.

Smoking: If either of you smoke, now is the time to quit. Talk to your doctors about options available to help you. Secondhand smoke is not only bad for the baby, but according to Getasthmahelp.org: "The exposure of secondhand smoke has been linked with many bad health effects, including cancers, heart disease, sudden infant death syndrome, middle ear problems and respiratory conditions." They also have a list of known health effects of secondhand smoke for infants and children. These include:

- Secondhand smoke has been shown to cause children to develop asthma.
- Infants who are exposed to secondhand smoke

have a higher risk of SIDS (Sudden Infant Death Syndrome), which is the leading cause of infant deaths from birth up to one year of age.
- Secondhand smoke also has been shown to cause low birth weights or babies to be too small for their gestational ages.

Of course, these are just a few of the problems that it can cause and I'm sure you don't want to worry about any of this while taking care of your pregnant partner. While I may be preaching to the choir here, I wanted to make sure to put this in the book. If it helps just one person quit smoking, then it's worth it.

Wine and beer: There is no research out there that wine or beer is good for the baby. In fact, according to Jacques Mortiz, MD, director of gynecology at St. Luke's-Roosevelt Hospital in New York, "The problem with drinking alcohol during your pregnancy is that there is no amount that has been proven to be safe."

You may hear friends and family say that they had a beer or a glass of wine here and there throughout their pregnancies and their kids are fine, but others will balk, saying this is just a risk that they never want to take. Pregnancies vary from woman to woman, and no two are exactly alike. Some women will have higher or lower enzymes that are able to break down alcohol in their bodies, which means that they could harm their baby with just one drink. Dr. David Garry, DO, associate professor of clinical obstetrics and gynecology at the Albert Einstein College of Medicine and chair of the Fetal Alcohol Spectrum Disorders Task Force for the American Collect of Obstetricians and Gynecologists District II/NY states, "If a pregnant woman with low levels of this enzyme drinks, her baby may be more susceptible to harm because the alcohol may circulate in her body for a longer period of time."

Bottom line – don't risk it. Don't let her risk it either.

At the end of this chapter, I've included some alternative 'mocktails' that you can fix for her if she has the craving for an alcoholic beverage.

Prenatal vitamins: If she has already gone to her doctor and picked up prenatal vitamins, great! If not, now is the time to call the doctor or pick up some at the local drug store. I will warn you, these are all huge pills and can look a little daunting. If she cannot take such large pills due to morning sickness, ask her doctor what other options are available.

Exercise: Now is the time to start an exercise routine. Walking is a great way to exercise and for you two to spend some time together talking without distractions. Her doctor can also recommend some exercises to do. Overall, it will help her if you're exercising with her to keep her motivated. Starting a plan now will make it easier to do along the way. Most doctors recommend 20-30 minutes of exercise per day if possible. Sometimes, she will be so sick or just miserable, that isn't in the cards. During those times, be supportive and find something else that you two can do together.

Help with morning sickness: Just offering crackers isn't enough. Help her through morning sickness as much as you can. This means to grab seasickness bracelets, holding her hair back, getting cool washcloths, ice packs and more. Anything that you can do to make this easier on her will help so much.

Nice things to do for your partner this month:

Here are some nice things that you can do for your partner this first month to show your excitement and your support:

Don't freak: When she tells you that she's pregnant, don't freak out. Be happy.

Flowers and gifts: Send her flowers or a delivered gift with a sweet card. While it sounds like a small, cliché thing, women love to be pampered and have gifts delivered, especially at work. It shows that you care and that you want everyone to know she's special.

Take her out to a nice dinner to celebrate: Here is the catch with this one, some women begin to have food turn offs right away. My wife could walk into a restaurant and immediately know if she could eat there or not without being sick. I can't tell you how many places we walked out of like a revolving door as soon as she smelled food. So, if you have to go to a few different places, be supportive. This is an issue that will bother her constantly, especially if she can no longer eat at her favorite place.

Surprise her with something special: When I say this, I don't mean a ring or a new car. I mean something simple, such as buying a funny onesie that she will like, picking up a cute pair of baby boots or sandals (make sure they are gender neutral since you won't have a clue what it will be yet), or taking her to look at paint swatches to start picking out nursery colors. Any small detail that you can do together now will make her happy and help both of your excitement grow.

Start doing dinner at least one night a week: Right now, this can be cooking dinner or picking up something that she wants. You want to get in the habit of doing this now, as chances are that you'll be cooking for yourself as morning sickness kicks in. (Note: morning sickness isn't just in the morning. It can last all day, every day.)

Easy dad recipes to make:

As I mentioned before, I have a few tricks up my sleeve when it comes to quenching that craving for alcoholic drinks. Here are a few recipes for mocktails that you can fix her while pregnant:

Mojito: Softly muddle (smash) mint leaves together and put them in the bottom of a glass. Then pour in half a teaspoon of lime juice, a teaspoon of simple syrup, and top with club soda. Stir and serve.

Fake champagne: Stir together one pgart pineapple juice, two parts white grape juice and three parts ginger ale. You can easily alter the portions of one ingredient to her liking.

Ginger Mule: Put ice and a few slices of cucumber in a glass. Then stir together ginger beer (make sure you get the non-alcoholic type) and a squeeze of fresh lime juice.

Watermelon Freeze: Mix watermelon, ice, honey and a small bit of sprite or club soda (a teaspoon or so) in a blender and serve. *This is a great summer pregnancy drink.

If you're stuck on what to make, ask what she would like to eat. Sometimes this will only be crackers and sprite, and you'll have to make due. If she is too sick to eat, I recommend against any food that has a potent smell. (You'll thank me later.) No matter if you're craving it or not, remember that she is fighting nausea over everything.

**NOTE: This advice is something that you will want to follow throughout the whole pregnancy as nausea will continue throughout the first trimester and sometimes beyond.

Make a list of food delivery services in your area, what type of food they offer, and their phone numbers to keep by the phone for nights when neither of you feel like cooking.

I also recommend that you learn some of her favorite foods and snacks so that you can have them stocked up for the times when she's famished. Of course, these probably will change throughout the pregnancy as her cravings come and go. So, you can't be too upset when she changes from craving honeydew melon to Nutella and pickles.

Chapter 2: Rolling Right Along

The second month

By now, the doctor has confirmed that yes, she is pregnant! It is fully time to celebrate. I'm sure you may have kept the news under wraps and you should make the decision together on who to tell and when to tell them. Don't let it slip to someone before you two have spoken about it. Chances are that you've probably already talked about it by now and have started telling people. If not, don't worry. There is no right or wrong time to say anything.

What's up with your partner

This is the month that she will start to experience some major changes in her body and moods. One of the first things to change will be her breasts. Most women experience tenderness and swelling and it will be no picnic for you, trust me. Sometimes even the slightest touch can bring her to tears, so make sure that you are careful if she mentions that they are tender. If she hasn't already gone shopping, take her, or give her a gift card or your credit card, and encourage her to buy some extra supportive, soft bras. Some women will actually grow a full cup size in the first few weeks.

Of course, you may, or may not, feel comfortable about talking with her about these things. If not, don't worry. You can always write a short, sweet note about it and surprise her with some cash and shopping time.

If she hasn't already felt the upset of morning sickness, this will be the month that it rears its ugly head. Its estimated that three out of four women suffer from this horrible symptom during their pregnancy. Here's the problem: that feeling can strike anywhere, anytime. There is no 'just mornings' about this problem so you also want to be ready to help her when she needs it, leave a restaurant before you've eaten, stop the car repeatedly and so on. Usually this starts sometime between the 4th to 9th week and will be at its worst sometime between the 7th and 12th weeks. As I mentioned in the first chapter, if this is bothersome or extreme, (or just plain horrible), call her doctor. There are so many options available to help her out.

During this time, her sense of smell will also become superwoman strength and she will notice everything. So, don't try to hide your gym bag in the other room, she'll smell it. Don't try to sneak a cigar in the garage, she'll smell it. Believe me, there were a lot of things that I wouldn't have thought she could have smelled when my wife was pregnant – but she did. This super smell power will also mean that there are certain foods she won't be able to even go around. For example, during her second pregnancy, my wife couldn't handle hamburgers cooking. Even when the neighbors two houses down from us grilled out, she got sick. However, her third pregnancy, she could handle hamburgers, but not bacon and eggs – and bacon is one of her all-time favorite foods. She even tried to force herself to eat her beloved bacon, but that wasn't a good idea, let me tell you.

One thing that almost always helped my wife were crackers of all types. Saltines mainly, but sometimes other crackers would work as well. If your partner is sick to the point they can't hold anything down, try to encourage her to eat some crackers – even if it's just a nibble here and there. Grab several boxes of the ones that she likes and stash sleeves of them here and there so she always has some handy. I made sure there were some on her nightstand, by the couch, on our patio (in the summer when we were out there a lot), in the car and several other places. Aside from helping her keep food down, the starchiness of the crackers can help take that edge of the nauseated feeling so she can try to eat more.

Along with the crackers, I also recommend that you find out which of the following she can handle during her pregnancy and keep it stocked as well: Sprite/Lemon-Lime soda, Ginger Ale, Gatorade (make sure you know what flavors), sparkling water or flavored waters. All of these can help keep her hydrated and also will help those crackers go down easier.

She also may start to have "pregnancy brain", which is just a fuzzy issue with memory and thinking. It's nothing serious and will come and go throughout the next few months. If it seems to be causing problems, buy her a small notebook that she can make lists or write important things down. Also download a good reminder or 'to do' app on her phone and help her put things in it so they are there to remind her of important things. My wife loved the app since she never went anywhere without her phone, even in the bathroom.

What's up with the peanut:

Beginning in the second month, (around week 5), your little peanut still isn't quite in a human form. Instead, it looks as if it still has tubes running everywhere. These tubes are forming into two vital organs: the brain and spinal cord and the heart. It also is starting to develop the tiny nubs that will become arms.

Around week six, something AMAZING happens: your baby's heart starts to beat! The teeny heart that beats is sitting in a tiny embryo about a half an inch long from it's head to it's rear. In fact, it's tiny little rear is about the size of a pencil eraser. More human-like features are beginning to form, such as eye lids, lungs, digestive organs and other vital organs that will help your baby start eating and breathing.

The kiddo is also attached to mommy by an umbilical cord. It's this connection that will provide everything the baby needs to grow so it can make a grand entrance.

What's Up With You:

I'm sure that the excitement is still bubbling over with the news, but chances are that there's a little hesitation and anxiety creeping in too. You're starting to worry about your partner, worrying if she's too sick or too forgetful or not eating enough… I could go on, but you already know. You're also starting to make mental lists of everything that you have to get done over the next few months and it's overwhelming. Trust me, I know. The best thing that you can do is to make a list. Use that coveted notebook or start a list of your own so that you can have it with you. Chop the list into parts, like to do today, to do this week, to do this month, to do in X number of months, etc.

Having small goals that you can cross off every day will help show you that you are accomplishing something. It also will help as you reach larger goals to see that you're not overwhelmed because you've planned out your list and you're following it.

Overall, take time to make sure that you are good. By this, I mean have a few minutes every day just to stop and breathe and remember that tiny little peanut that will make its entrance in just a few short months.

Key things to do this month:

Now that everything is rolling along, there are some things that you need to do:

Stick to foods that appeal to her: This one should be self-explanatory. Prepare foods that she wants to eat, even if it's only crackers. Don't branch out and decide this is the month to learn to make sushi. It won't end well. Her tastes might change from week to week – or even day to day, but you want to keep track and pay attention so you don't accidentally set off something that keeps her from eating for a day or more.

Help her remember to eat: I know, this sounds stupid, but it's not. You need to make sure that she's eating something right when she wakes up and right before she goes to bed – even if its crackers. Having something in her tummy will help with the nausea. You also want to remind her to just graze on food throughout the day. She doesn't have to gorge herself every meal, but she doesn't need to go for hours on empty either. That is one of the worst things to do when morning sickness is hitting hard. Having something in her stomach constantly will help fight the nausea.

Fluids are key: No matter what, you have to make sure that she is staying hydrated. This is why I mentioned earlier that you needed to stock up on whatever she felt like drinking. Have these things around constantly so there is always something there for her to drink. If she gets dehydrated, it can really make nausea worse and it can cause serious problems that mean a trip to the ER if you're not careful.

Relaxation is a must: No matter how busy your days are, make time to allow her to just relax. It can be just a nap or time in a bubble bath or a trip to get her nails done, it doesn't matter what it is. Just make sure that she takes a few moments to relax and destress a bit. It will help her and the baby – and you as well.

Oral hygiene: Along with the fun of nausea and all that goes with it, she needs to brush her teeth after any time she vomits or eats. Of course, let her tummy settle a bit first. If her normal toothpaste is causing some of the issues with nausea, try several different brands until there is one that doesn't immediately cause that green-faced monster to come out. Her doctor can also recommend a good rinse or toothpaste if you can't find one.

Baby registry: She may have already been working on this, but you should offer to help. Sometimes it's fun just for the two of you to go 'window shopping' for items that you'd like to have for the baby. Create a registry at several different places because you never know what stores are near your family and friends when they head out shopping. Make sure that you also include items you'll need a lot of, such as onesies, blankets, burp cloths and so on.

Nice things to do for your partner this month:

Paid for relaxation: Buy her a gift card to get her nails done, a pedicure, a massage (there are practitioners who only do pregnant massage and they are amazing!), or something else that she loves to do that will relax her.

Can you say 'more pillows': Body pillows will help her sleep better, especially if you can find the overstuffed ones. Buy a couple because later on, she'll have to sleep propped up on them in weird positions so the baby doesn't jump on her bladder all night.

Keep up the good deeds: Remember all those 'nice things' I recommended for the first month? (If not, they are still there if you need a reminder.) Continue to do these things for her. Don't just do a few one month and stop. The happier and more relaxed she is, the easier the pregnancy will be on you both. Plus, it will help her self-esteem as the pregnancy goes on to know that you still see that beautiful woman you married, even if she doesn't feel like her anymore.

Read pregnancy books, articles and more: The more than you can learn about what she's going through, the better you'll understand it and be able to help. I mean, hey, you've already picked up this book – so that's a start. There are thousands of great pieces out there that will help you know what to do.

Easy dad recipes to make:

I gave you some good drink recipes in the first chapter, so now, let's go over a few throw-it-together-in-five-minutes recipes for those times you forgot to order something!

Spaghetti: Ok guys, if you don't know how to make spaghetti, you seriously need to get online and watch some youtube videos. All kidding aside, this is one of the easiest things that you can throw together for you or the kiddos on nights where dinner happens in that 'panic mode'. (You know, where everyone is frazzled from the day, it's 7:45 and the kids are fighting, they still need baths, their homework finished, the dog needs to go out repeatedly, your wife is stuck in the bathroom and you still have to feed everyone. Yeah, those are spaghetti nights. It is beyond simple to make: you get a package of spaghetti noodles (or fettuccini, angel hair, etc) and boil it in a pot of water until the noodles are tender. Pop open a jar of your favorite spaghetti sauce into a pan and warm it up. Drain the noodles, pour them and the sauce back into the large pot or a large bowl, and bam. Dinner.

Easy grilled cheese: All this consists of is bread, butter, and cheese. The key to great grilled cheese sandwiches is to butter the sides of the bread that are going to touch the griddle. Place one buttered bread side down on the griddle/frying pan/etc, add a slice of cheese, then place the other buttered side up on top of the cheese. Now when it's ready to flip, you'll be flipping the other buttered side down. The key is to make sure you have the temperature down low enough that it won't sear the bread to a beautiful black right away. You want golden brown bread.

Insane scrambled eggs: (This is a name my kids came up with for the scrambled eggs that I made them a lot when my wife was pregnant.) You'll need eggs, shredded cheese, and bacon strips or bits, ham chunks, or any other meats (precooked) you want to add, and black olives or tomatoes (or both). All you do is spray down your pan with non-stick spray and turn the heat on medium. Crack 2 eggs per person into a bowl, add a tiny bit of water, salt, and pepper and mix with a fork until it's all one yellowy goo. Pour the mix into the frying pan and let it sit for a bit. You'll know when to start scraping them around with the spatula when you can see some of the eggs are starting to become hard as they cook. Stir/scrape/flip the cooked egg parts around until they start to form a fluffy mush. Once the eggs are just about all finished (i.e. no liquidy areas), when you sprinkle in a bunch of shredded cheese, your meats, and vegetables. You shouldn't have to do more than just melt the cheese. You'll then have a gooey meaty mess that tastes amazing.

*TIP: if you have little kids – or big kids too – you can add in a couple of drops of food coloring to turn your eggs different colors. Just remember that they are yellow, so that will affect the color you're going for. For example, if you want green eggs, add in some blue (not too much). When I made green eggs, my kids called them alien eggs.

Variation on insane eggs: If you don't want to stand over the stove, here's an easy way to make insane eggs in the microwave. Mix up the mix as I listed above with one small difference: you want to cook the eggs in batches of 3 to 4 each. Pour this mix into a microwave safe bowl and set on high for 3 to 4 minutes. The kids will like to watch this, as the eggs puff up, and almost overwhelm the bowl. You want to check and make sure there are no liquid parts after the time is up. Add in the cheese and other items and microwave for about 30 seconds to a minute so the cheese is melted.

Then you can throw them on a plate and serve! (We call these 'space eggs' at my house.)

Chapter 3: Finishing Up the First Trimester

The third month:

Doctors' visits pick up at this point and depending on how your partner is doing, you may be going once every month or every week. If you can, go to every doctors' appointment with her. This is not just for moral support, but it will also help you be involved with decisions and ask questions that she might not think to ask. Plus, you can take the coveted notebook and make sure all of your questions are answered and write down important information.

On top of that, you won't miss things like: hearing the heartbeat for the first time, seeing the peanut (if the doctor does an ultrasound that early), and so on. I will tell you that hearing that heartbeat for the very first time will completely change your world!

This is also the month when the doctor should be doing all sorts of tests, if they haven't already. These will include gestational diabetes, ultrasounds, alpha-fetoprotein tests or multiple marker tests, chorionic villus sampling and amniocentesis. These tests are done in the first trimester to ensure there are no problems or needs that the doctor needs to treat during the pregnancy. While your doctor may require other tests, here is a breakdown of the normal testing done this month:

Gestational diabetes: This is a one hour initial test to check how glucose is taken care of in the mother's body. They have her drink a very thick, syrupy mix – that apparently tastes horrible, just a warning – and then they can tell if the mother's body is or isn't tolerating the glucose well. If she isn't, they will do other tests and probably put her on a diet for diabetics to ensure that she nor the baby will have issues during and after birth.

Ultrasound: Pretty much everyone knows about the ultrasound! This is where you get to finally see your peanut for the first time. Usually, you can learn the sex of the baby if you would like. But this test also checks for abnormalities with the baby's growth – and for multiple kiddos in there. Depending on the mother's age as well as any health issues during pregnancy, you may have just one ultrasound, or multiple ones.

Alpha-fetoprotein or multiple marker: This tests for a protein produced in the fetal liver and is in the amniotic fluid. The protein also crosses over the placenta into the mother's blood. The AFP levels can signal the following problems: open neural tube defects (like spina bifida), down syndrome, defects in the abdominal wall of the fetus, twins!, miscalculated due date, and other chromosomal abnormalities.

Chorionic villus: This is a test sometimes called CVS that takes some of the placental tissue and shows if there are chromosomal abnormalities that may need further testing or if there are any other genetic problems. The test will also be done if there is a history of genetic defects or disorders in the family history.

Amniocentesis: This test is normally done if there are abnormal readings in the AFP tests, if she is over 35, if there was an abnormal maternal serum screening, increased risk for chromosomal abnormalities or tube defects, to check if both babies are healthy if there are multiple babies or if they need to make sure that the baby is growing properly and ok to be delivered. (The last part of that, the growing properly, is usually later in the pregnancy if she has gone into early labor and they either cannot stop it or it keeps happening.) I won't lie, it's a scary looking test with a huge needle. My wife had it done and did say that it hurt, however, we were more worried about how our little one was growing since she had gone into early labor three times.

Group B streptococcus (GBS): This strain of strep is found in the lower genital area of around 25% of women. It doesn't cause any normal problems;

however it can cause serious illness during pregnancy. This also can cause life-threatening infections with the baby when it's born, like meningitis and pneumonia.

WHAT'S UP WITH YOUR PARTNER:

If she hasn't already had issues with her breasts being sore, now is the month that starts to get worse. These changes will continue to get worse until around the end of the first trimester (the third month), but can stick around for the remainder of the pregnancy. The girls will be full and heavy and sore and it will make her miserable at times. Make sure that you ask if there is anything at all that you can do for her and don't blow off weird or small requests. Do anything that she thinks may help. Hopefully, they will stop hurting after this month, even if they continue to grow.

You may notice that she is sleeping a lot and seriously tired when she isn't sleeping. Right now, her body is working beyond overtime. She's creating the placenta, which is the life support system for the peanut. Don't get offended or be mad that she's taking another nap, or that she missed this show with you or made you guys late to a dinner party. Besides, if you are late somewhere, no one will be mad at a pregnant lady! (Trust me!)

What's up with the peanut:

Here's where things start to get fun! That tiny thing now weighs about the same as a penny, around 1/8 of an ounce. It has replaced that tiny tail looking appendage with two amazing legs. While it's noggin is still massive for the rest of its body, all of that will even out as the baby grows. The webbing between its toes and fingers are gone, it's eyes are wide open right now (even though they will close again temporarily in a bit),

Here is something truly amazing: during this month, your baby's reproductive organs have developed already! While you won't be able to tell on the ultrasound (if you have one at this point), you may see the baby move. It's amazing that at this early stage, it's reproductive organs have already been formed.

What's up with you:

If you've been going to doctors' appointments, then you may be over the moon at this point. If you haven't, don't worry. You may also be helping pick out cribs and other necessity items, as well as helping create a gift registry for the baby shower. Seeing these items in your home will really help make things even more real for you and more exciting. If you've been keeping up with your list, you're starting to see things crossed off and that list getting shorter. Make sure that you're adding to it as you go along so that you don't miss anything important and remember at the last minute.

Key things to do this month:

Steer clear of the tatas: During sex, be careful not to grab them too hard or anything that can cause discomfort. Yes, I know, this can screw up your game if you're worried about that. However, if they cause her to scream in pain, then playtime is over.

It's the hormones talking – really: She went from wonderful, fluttery, happy to insane Linda Blair spewing pea soup in the form of foul words in less than ten seconds. What the hell did you say or do? You are now so confused it's not even remotely funny and you're quickly rolling everything through your mind to see what you said or did. Let me stop you right there: chances are that it's hormones and mood swings doing the talking. Unless you two have just been in a knock down drag out fight, which I don't recommend, then you're probably on the receiving end of a mood swing. Don't worry. It will pass. Soon, she'll either be beyond sorry or she will be in the bathroom crying because a tissue ripped. Try not to snap back at her and resist the urge to say something like "Why are you crying now?" or "What's the matter with you?" Yeah, those don't end well. Just remember that hormones are really taking a toll on her and sometimes a long hug and a kiss on the forehead are the best remedy.

Car seat time: If you two haven't already been looking at car seats to take the baby home in, now is the time to start. There are so many great brands and styles out there it should be easy to find one you both like. Keep in mind that they can be a bit expensive, so be prepared. Also, you want to make sure that you find a seat that has a base that snaps onto the carrier. This will make things so much easier on you when taking the little peanut out of the house. Plus, the hospital won't let you leave with the baby until they know you have a safe car seat for him or her.

Nice things to do for your partner this month:

She may be starting to show at this point and she also may be exhausted and sore from the major changes in her body. So look for ways that you can help around the house with things that she normally does:

Vacuuming and mopping: These are activities that she really doesn't need to be doing as it can put some strain on those already sore stomach muscles. If you can take care of this chore, she will love you for it. (Just don't run the vacuum while she's asleep!)

Cleaning: Along with that first point, any cleaning that you can do will help as well. Keep in mind that cleaning product fumes may make her sick – and she doesn't need to be using bleach either.

Snack delivery: If there is something she's craving, offer to go to the store and pick it up for her. You may also see if there's a grocery list that you can take care of as well.

Step up your help with older children if you have them: By helping get older kids ready for school, helping with homework, fixing afterschool snacks and so on, you can help her out by taking that worry off her plate.

Take maternity photos: This is one thing that we have done through every pregnancy and made a collage out of it to frame. It is fun to take photos throughout her pregnancy and see how far the baby decides to push out (ever baby is carried a little differently believe it or not) and to see how fast the baby grows.

Stay away from deleting shows on your DVR: I made the mistake of deleting some shows she'd already watched and paid the price for it. If she has a favorite show, just leave those episodes there for her to watch again when insomnia strikes. If you find a show or movie you think she'll enjoy, record it and let her know about it. You never know when she'll need something to watch late at night.

Easy Dad Recipes to Make:

Need some more easy fix things for you and the kids (if you already have kids)? Here are a few of my other favorites:

Quesadillas: They are easier to make than you think. All you really need is tortillas and cheese. However, you can add in whatever meats or veggies you like. Here is what you do: heat up a griddle or frying pan to almost medium heat. If you have a gas range, low is good. Lay a tortilla down and spread cheese and other toppings on one side of the tortilla. Then use a spatula to pull the unfilled side of the tortilla over on top of the filled side. Cook on the filled side until the cheese it melted and holding both sides of the tortilla together. Carefully flip over with the spatula and cook for a minute or so until the bottom is a golden brown. Cut into thirds or fourths and serve.

Sloppy Joes: Ok, this has to be one of the easiest things ever to make. Head to the store and grab hamburger buns and a couple of cans of sloppy joe mix. There are so many different flavors and variations of sloppy joe mix that you can easily find one that everyone will like. Heat up the contents of the can either on the stove in a pot or in the microwave and spread a large spoonful onto a hamburger bun. Serve and you're done!

Pancakes: Here is another one that's so simple. At the store, pick up butter, syrup and pancake mix. Bisquick is my personal favorite, but there are tons of different types out there. Make sure that you have eggs and oil if the mixing instructions on the box call for them. Mix the ingredients according to the directions on the box, and pour by spoonfuls onto a hot griddle. I usually leave the heat down to right at the low/medium line. If you have gas, you may want to go a little lower. Let the pancakes sit until there are unbroken bubbles on the top. Then carefully flip. Leave it there for a minute or so and reflip to check the bottom. When both sides are golden, they're ready.

Chapter 4: The Second Trimester

The fourth month:

During this month, she may really be starting to show a good-sized bump. Chances are that she's either self-conscious or ecstatic about it. She is supposed to gain weight, so let her know that nicely if she complains, blame it on the peanut needing nourishment or jokingly talk about how the little kiddo is craving x or y and needs more of it. Never say she's gaining too much weight, even if you say it jokingly. Her doctor will be the one to address that and then you won't have to be the bad guy!

If you haven't learned yet what the sex of the baby is, this month it should be easier for the doctor to tell. So, if you want to know, make sure to ask.

What's up with your partner:

Beginning around the fourth month, she has a ton of things on her mind. She may not be sleeping well as the peanut will be awake most of the night. Her girlfriends may also be wearing her out. And she may still be extremely sick all day, every day. Forgive her for snapping at you over a tiny thing. Make sure to hug her and reassure her that she is still as beautiful as the day you met, except now she's glowing. Hearing reassurances will help her self-esteem as the baby bump grows and other pregnancy related health issues pop up.

She may also be noticing some stretch marks at this point, which can go one of two ways: she can blow them off and wear them as a badge of motherhood or... she can start a long, sobbing cry about how they are ruining her body. Either way, reassure her they make no difference to you and that you look at them as a heroic badge that men can never earn. (Seriously, phrase it in that tone to flatter her strength and the wonder of birth and it will help that conversation immediately.)

WHAT'S UP WITH THE PEANUT:

While the little munchkin is only about four to five inches long now about the size of a small cell phone – not one of those huge screened monsters – there's still a lot going on. At this point, your baby has kidneys that are producing urine. Also, you can see a cute little peek of thumb sucking on an ultrasound as the beginning of this month is when most babies discover they can suck on their own thumb. Your kiddo can also see light that filters in from outside, even though it's eyelids are still firmly shut.

If she hasn't felt the baby move yet, this is the month most that will start and it will be extremely exciting! One thing that we loved on ultrasounds was to see the baby moving, we got to see a facial expression change, and we even saw our daughter blink – which surprised our doctor.

Your baby also is now covered in tiny soft hair, much like peach fuzz. It's called lanugo and provides a little coat of sorts in the womb. The kiddo is also developing hair on it's head, eyelashes, and eyebrows. There is an old wives' tale that the more hair a baby has, the worse heartburn will be on the mother. My wife swears by this as well, however, I'm not too sure.

During this month, the tiny ears have developed enough to hear your voices, so talk to the baby as much as possible.

Here is something that I still think is extremely cool: at this point, your baby is developing its own set of fingerprints during this month.

What's Up With You:

Find yourself working too much? Finding reasons to work overtime? Working your rear off outside or in the garage? It's normal for some dads to overcompensate because they feel they are uninvolved in the massive baby craze with the family. Yes, it is the women who will dote on your wife more and she will also be getting most of the attention. However, don't worry. If you do feel uninvolved, as I mentioned before, talk to your partner and nicely address your feelings. Volunteer to go with her to run errands, help put away baby gifts, help plan the shower and other things. Ensure you're well involved without being overpowering.

Your partner also may not even realize she has been leaving you out of things. So, opening a good line of positive communication will do wonders to fix this problem. Remember the 'positive' part of this because her emotions will be all over the place and you don't want to make the problem worse with the wrong wording.

On the other hand, she may feel that she's already burning you out talking about baby stuff. If you assure her that could never happen, she's more likely to truly burn you out on the subject – just in a good way.

Here is the problem with working too much: if your relationship is already strained a bit from stress or other issues, being overworked and never at home will only cause this rift to grow. In turn, that will cause more problems with you feeling uninvolved, problems in the bedroom and problems with normal communication.

Key things to do this month:

There are a few things that you need to make sure to take care of or start the process on:

Family leave: Check with your HR department at work to see what the Family Leave policy entails. You may only have a couple of days or a week or more. Either way, you need to know how long it is, what you need to do to take it when the baby comes and any other important details.

Vacation: This is also a good time to check and see

how much vacation time you have built up and how much you will have around the due date. You also need to know how to request vacation time after the family leave time is up. If you start working on this now, you won't have any unexpected snags when the kiddo arrives.

Names, names and more names: If you haven't already started chatting about names for the baby (which I'm sure you have at this point), now is the time to start narrowing down the search. If there are issues with naming the baby after a family member on one side or the other, try combining names to please you both. For example, if your dad's name is Robert and her dad's name is Michael, you can easily use Michael Robert (or the other way around). It's pretty easy if you write their names down and see which way you can combine them.

Learn to handle frequent bathroom stops: Yes, they get annoying to you but imaging how she feels having to pee every five minutes. These stops will only continue as the pregnancy goes on, so learn to either add extra time to trips or just deal with them when they pop up.

Nice things to do for your partner this month:

Of course, I still recommend continuing the other nice things I've already listed in previous chapters; but here are some more:

Baby name ideas: Even if you've both talked about names until you're blue in the face, chances are that you may not be set on a specific name yet. Here's a nice thing that will mean a lot to her: go out and buy a couple of baby name books and search the web for several sites that offer names and their meanings, then bookmark them. Set up a special 'date' where you can fix her favorite cravings and the two of you go through baby names uninterrupted. That means put the phones out of reach, turn off the tv, and wait until the kids are gone or in bed (if you already have munchkins).

Pregnancy massage: I know that I mentioned this before, however it is one thing that helped my wife more than anything. If you haven't already done this, shame on you! (Just kidding) Look online and see if there are any places that do pregnant massage. By now, your partner is stressed (usually in a good way), tired, has sore muscles and her back is starting to hurt from the weigh shifting more to the front as the baby grows. This massage is well worth the month and she will appreciate it more than you know. Make time for her to have one often if you can.

Tell her she is beautiful and you love her: There will be days that she feels like Gollum from Lord of the Rings and will be doing anything she can to hide herself. This is when she needs you most. Hug her and tell her that you love her more than anything and how beautiful she is. Just this small gesture can help make her whole day that much better. However, you don't have to just do it at those times. Do it every day so she never forgets it.

Easy dad recipes to make:

Here are several more easy fix recipes that you can try:

Pizza Pinwheels: Ok, we are getting to just a little bit more steps, but these are still easy. You'll need 1 8oz can of refrigerated pizza dough, 2 cups of shredded mozzarella cheese, a package of pepperoni, and a 14oz can of pizza sauce. Heat your oven to 375 degrees and spray your cooking sheet with non-stick spray. On the baking sheet, roll out the pizza dough and spread a layer of pizza sauce over the whole area of the dough. Then layer on the cheese and pepperonis. Roll the dough back up as tight as possible and then slide into pieces about an inch thick. Lay these pieces on the sheet so there is enough room for them to grow just a bit while cooking. Pop the sheet in the over for about 10-12 minutes until the tops are golden brown. Serve with or without pizza sauce!

Chicken and cheese: Another super easy one. You'll need chicken breasts or chicken tender meat, seasonings (salt, pepper, and lemon pepper if you wish) and your choice of shredded cheese. I personally use either the Fiesta Blend from Kraft or Colby jack. Preheat your oven to 375 and spray down your baking sheet (or cheat and use foil for easy clean up). Cut the chicken breasts into almost bite sized pieces and sprinkle with your desired amount of seasonings. Pop these guys in the oven and cook for about 15 minutes or until the chicken is cooked all the way through. (If you aren't sure how to tell if the chicken is cooked, simply pull off the thickest piece and cut in half. If it's solid white, it's good. If there is still some pink, pop it back in the oven.) Once the chicken is done, spread a layer of cheese on top of every piece of chicken. Turn your oven off then put the baking sheet back in the oven so the cheese can melt without getting scorched. Serve and enjoy!

Tater tot taco casserole: You'll need 1 pound of ground beef, 1 package taco seasoning mix, 1 16oz bag of frozen Mexican style corn, 1 12oz can of black beans (rinsed and drained), 1 12oz bag of shredded Mexican cheese blend, 1 16oz package of frozen tater tots, 1 12oz can of enchilada sauce, and 1 small diced onion (if you like onions). Heat the oven to 375 degrees and spray down a 9x13 inch baking dish. Cook the ground beef in a skillet over a medium heat, stirring the meat around until it's all browned. Drain the grease off of the meat (NOT in the sink, in a empty glass container) and add in the beans, the corn, the taco seasoning, and the onion and cook slightly. Set aside to cool a bit. Then mix the ground beef mix and the tater tots and ¾ of the bag of cheese in a large bowl and stir until the tater tots are coated. Pour about 1/3 of the enchilada sauce into the baking dish and then spoon in the tater tot mix. You may have to pat the mix down to get a solid and even layer. Pour the remaining enchilada sauce on top of that. Bake in the oven for about 40 minutes. When it's finished, turn the oven off and put the remaining cheese on top. Put it back in the oven so the cheese can melt. Let cool and serve!

Chapter 5: The Halfway Mark

The fifth month

You've made it to the halfway mark in the pregnancy and it can seem like the time is going too fast one day, then too slow the next. There is a lot to do to get prepared for that little bundle of joy and you need to start preparing now.

What's up with your partner:

During this month, the doctor will begin to monitor your partner's weigh closer. In 2015, the CDC did a study that found about 47% of women in the US gain more than the recommended weight during pregnancy, which puts them at higher risks for problems. These problems happen during and after pregnancy, and could affect the health of both her and the baby. So, the doctor will make sure that she is keeping on the right track. However, about 1 in 5 moms gains too little weight or even loses some due to being so sick. The recommended amount of weight to gain is between 25 and 35 pounds which is gauged by her BMI (Body Mass Index). Basically, gradual weight gain is key.

Of course, if you two are lucky enough to have multiple babies, her doctor will go over weight gain and other issues to ensure that all the babies will be healthy and happy.

That scale in your bathroom will become a hated thing. Doctors and experts all recommend that pregnant women take the following tips to heart when it comes to weighing themselves during pregnancy:

- Weigh at the same time of day, not in the morning one time and then after a huge lunch the next
- Wear the same amount of clothing each time, or just your undies if possible
- Use the same scale, don't switch it up by buying a new one halfway through
- Only weigh yourself once a week or you'll go crazy with the liquid fluctuations and other differences in your day to day meals

I understand the obsession with weighing yourself, as my wife did it way too much with our first kid. By the second one, she hated that scale and only had her weight checked at the doctor's office. Her doctor recommended weighing herself once a week to keep track of weight gain and see any issues when they start, not when it's too late.

What's up with the peanut:

Man is that little thing growing like a weed at this point. Kiddo is about the size of a banana at this point and you can feel movements so much better when you lay your hands on her belly. The term for this is 'quickening' and I guarantee she knows this term and has been waiting for it to begin. You may hear the doctor use this term or 'fetal movement' and it's just like it sounds: the baby's movements can be felt outside the womb. At first, she may be the only one who can feel them, but don't wo

If you have started talking to the baby, which I am sure you have, you may notice that it responds to your voice at times.

Along with the thin layer of hair that has grown in the last month, your baby is also developing a waxy substance on its body called vernix caseosa. This wax is formed to help the baby's delicate skin as the amniotic fluid can irritate it, even though it is helping the baby grow. It is kind of a weird trade off. Your baby's hair will really be growing at this point and your partner is enjoying perks from this as well since her hair is growing in thicker too.

Your kiddo also has tiny tooth buds growing under its gums and the bone marrow is kicking its red blood production into high gear. These red blood cells will deliver oxygen to the baby after its born.

Inside that tiny body, the intestines are starting to produce meconium, which are the weird looking, tarry, sticky waste that you'll see in those first few diapers.

What's Up With You:

Chances are that you are starting to realize it's getting closer to that big day when you finally get to meet baby. You also may have heard some horror stories of other pregnancies at this point and have small panic attacks when you think something could happen to your wife or baby. Remember that her doctor is monitoring everything and if there are issues, you will know immediately and the doctor will be taking steps to fix them.

You also might be having some second thoughts about this whole baby thing. Worried about what kind of dad you'll be, have no idea what the doctor was trying to say yesterday, constantly thinking about every little thing she does and how it affects the baby and… well, you get the drift. Let me tell you right now, everyone goes through this. I did. With every pregnancy. So, don't worry about worrying. It will pass, I promise. Once you see that tiny face and hear that first cry, nothing else will matter.

However, I also recommend talking to your partner as well. I almost guarantee you that she's been thinking the same things you have. Make some time to have a freak out together about the whole situation and then get it off your chests. It will make both of you feel better. Just remember that parents have been raising kids since the dawn of time. It is easier than you think.

Key things to do this month:

There are several things that you need to do this month to help both her and you keep everything running smoothly:

Calories are key: Making sure that she is getting the right number of calories for a healthy pregnancy is key to a healthy baby and mama. Of course, this can be hard when cravings can fluctuate so wildly during a pregnancy. Her doctor will probably tell you guys that during this second trimester, she should be adding about 300 more calories per day and during the third trimester, bump that up to 500. This is easier said than done, so try to help her stay as close to that as possible without micromanaging her diet. Toward the end of this book, you'll find a list of great foods to eat while pregnant to help her pick some items that she loves that will help her too.

Birth plan: If she hasn't already started thinking about a birth plan, now is the time to start. In no way is this something that can wait until the last minute as you have to have doctors picked out, preparations made and so on. A birth plan is a detailed description of how she wants her labor and delivery to go. This will include: who she wants in the room, how she wants to go into labor *hopefully*, what your role will be, what doctor she is using, who may be on call if that doctor is not available, what pediatrician you guys intend to use and more. Keep in mind that this is an ideal plan of what she'd like, however, things can go haywire so this is not set in stone.

Birthing classes: If this is your first kiddo, I highly recommend birthing classes. We did take them with our first child and they were a huge help. There is a lot of information online or you can check with the hospital that she will be delivering at and find out where local classes are. This is a fun thing that you two can to do together to get you more involved and have some time away from the house to learn happy things about the delivery.

Visit the hospital: You probably know what hospital she'll be delivering in and it's a great idea to take time to visit and find out where everything is. Trust me, you don't want to be heading up there after her water's broken, trying to figure out where to go! If you go visit well in advance – a few times – you'll have a firm grip on where to go, where to park, what elevator to take and so on. Knowing all of this ahead of time will help you stay calm while she isn't. Keep in mind that you'll be staying at the hospital from 24-48 hours after the baby is born, so you will also want to know where vending machines, the cafeteria, nurses' stations, maternity ward and the nursery are.

Nice things to do for your partner this month:

I hope that you're still doing all of the things from previous chapters to keep her, and you, happy. However, here are some more things that you can do for her:

Special baby gifts: Sure, she's getting all kinds of gifts and trinkets from everyone else, so why do you need to get her a baby gift too? I mean, it's your kid, right? Yes and no. I mean, yes, it's your kid; but no in the fact that you don't need to get her something. Here is what I recommend: find a small item and have it personalized for her. My favorite thing to do is to find the little plaster kits that allow you to make tiny hand and foot prints when your kiddo is born. I did this for every pregnancy and we have them lined up on our mantle. It is something intimate that just the two of you can do when you are finally home alone with the baby. Items like this, that you can personalize and do together make a huge difference and might even cause tears, the good kind.

Half way celebration: Plan a surprise date night with her to celebrate your 'half way pregnancy anniversary'. Buy her a new dress or something nice to wear, dress up a little and go somewhere she loves for dinner. Catch a movie. Goof off at a mall. Walk around a beautiful area near where you live like a park or lake. Just do something special, just the two of you. Also, make sure to buy her something special, a ring or necklace, something unique and not just a box of her favorite junior mints. Truly put some thought into it. I guarantee it will mean more to her than you know.

Easy dad recipes to make:

More easy dad recipes!

Bacon wrapped shrimp: You'll need 1 to 2 packages of bacon (I cheat and use the microwave kind that's already cooked), a package of medium sized shrimp precooked, and toothpicks. Preheat the oven to 325 Thaw the shrimp. If you get raw bacon, fry it first until it's firm but still bendable. If you get microwave bacon, it's already ready for the next step. Slice the bacon pieces in half. Take one shrimp and wrap a half a slice of bacon around it and put a toothpick through to hold it together. Place on a baking sheet. Continue to do this until all the shrimp are bacon wrapped and on the baking sheet. Pop in the oven for about 15 minutes, then let cool and serve!

Chicken chunk lollipops: This is a fun recipe for adults or kids! Here's what you'll need: 4 skinless boneless chicken breasts cut into ½ inch cubes, 1 egg, 2 tablespoons of milk, 2 cups of crushed potato chips (you can use the plain Lays or Ruffles or get creative and use sour cream and onion, barbeque or other flavors), and lollipop sticks from a craft or party store. If you can't find the sticks, you can use skewers and put several of chicken pieces on one skewer. Preheat the oven to 350 degrees and spray your baking sheet. Crush the potato chips on a plate until they are a pretty fine mess. You don't want to make them into a powder, just a good smashed up mix. Then mix together the water, egg and milk. Stir this mix with a whisk or a fork if you don't have a whisk. Then dip the chicken pieces into the water mix, coat it with the potato chips goodness and put onto the baking sheet. Continue until all chicken pieces are coated. Bake for 10 minutes, then carefully turn all of the nuggets over and bake another 10 minutes. When they are finished, let them cool just a bit and insert the lollipop stick or skewer into them and serve. *You can also set out several different types of dipping sauces in small bowls for an extra fun aspect.

Easy taco bake: Here's what you need for this crazy good dinner: 1 ½ pound lean ground beef, 1 package taco seasoning mix, 1 16oz can of refried beans, 1 16oz jar of salsa and 2 cups shredded Monterey Jack cheese. Heat the oven to 325 and spray down a 9x13 inch baking dish. Then brown the ground beef in a large skillet over medium-high heat and drain the fat off. Mix in the dry taco seasoning and stir. Spoon the meat into the baking dish. Then spoon in the refried beans (I find it's a little easier if you put them in a bowl and microwave them a bit to make them spread easier). Now spread the salsa over the beans and add the cheese to the top in a full layer. Bake at 325 for about 20-25 minutes.

Chapter 6: Growing Baby, Growing Belly

The sixth month:

The little ninja kicking you from inside her belly now weighs about one pound and is approximately eight inches from head to rear. Talk about growing! Toward the middle to end of this month, your child is grown enough that if the unthinkable happened and it had to be born now, it would more than likely survive with the help of a ventilator. So that should take one fear out of your head (hopefully).

Toward the end of this month, your kiddo will almost double in size and weigh about two pounds!

What's up with your partner:

If she hasn't noticed (or had any) stretch marks, now is the time that they will start to show more. Since baby is growing really rapidly and growing much bigger than normal skin stretches, these marks are bound to happen. However, these will fade after delivery. Every woman is different, so they could completely go away or they could remain dark purple for a long time. Make sure that you reassure her that they make her more beautiful.

Hormones start to ramp up as the baby gets bigger, so don't get too worked up if her mood swings really start fluctuating. This can make her extremely tired, really cranky, crying at every little thing or so many other variations that you could never list them all. Just relax and remember that it's the hormones talking, and she will more than likely apologize later.

What's up with the peanut:

At the start of this month, kiddo is forming into a full-fledged tiny human. It's systems and organs have all the material and genetic information on how to operate, how it's senses will work and so on. Its tiny lungs will get ready to breathe air by inhaling fluid. As the lungs do this, they are also producing something called surfactant, which allows its little lungs to inflate. It's also during this second week that the tiny brain is making the connections needed to think – so the kiddo will be ready to negotiate with you to get its way later!

While its tiny skin had been as wrinkly as a raisin, all those folds are starting to fill out as fatty layers build up underneath. Kiddo also now has the first bits of finger and toe nails. The skin also begins to go from see through to cloudy, the first signs of pigment in the epidermis.

You also may be able to press your ear against her belly and faintly hear a heartbeat or hiccups! While it finally has the eyelids completely formed, they are now open and underneath are beautiful bluish eyes. However, don't get too attached to those baby blues. It probably will change in the first few months.

What's up with you:

If there hasn't been a baby shower yet, it will probably happen in this last trimester. It's not just women that can go to these baby showers. Have a dad shower by grilling and inviting the other husbands over to hang out while the women are ogling gifts and giggling. Plus, if you're grilling food or even if you pick up food, it will help out with the shower foods instead of just sweets.

I'm also going to point out once again that you should remember that it is all about the baby. Sure, she will be getting most of the attention, but this isn't anything personal toward the dad – it just the facts. Don't let it get to you.

If you've noticed that you're gaining more weight as she does, it's normal. If it's bothersome to you, don't make a show out of it and simply do things that will help you shed those extra pounds. Trust me, you will gain more before the baby is here.

KEY THINGS TO DO THIS MONTH:

Hopefully, you've kept up with things I've mentioned here as well as items that the doctor has mentioned, such as different classes. If not, here are several things that you need to work on this month:

Phone numbers: If you don't already have her family and friend's phone numbers, you need to start gathering them. She may not want to sit and text or make calls after the baby gets here so this job will more than likely fall to you. If you're not a phone person, designate one friend or family member to make these calls for you after the baby gets here. This way, no one is left out when the news spreads about your bundle of joy.

Stocking up: While baby isn't here yet, it's always a great idea to start stocking up on diapers, wipes, powder, sanitizer, diaper cream, formula (if she doesn't plan to breast feed), snacks for her after baby is here, onsies and other items. You will never realize how fast diapers will disappear after kiddo comes home for the hospital.

Nice things to do for your partner this month:

Since she's got a growing belly at this point, it's always nice to help out and continue doing all of the things I've already mentioned. However, here are some others that will I suggest at this point:

Foot props: Around the sixth month is when her feet will start that wonderful swelling and she will be absolutely miserable. Find a way for her to relax with her feet propped up to help the swelling go down and to relax her in general. Sometimes this can by lying on the couch with her feet propped up on pillows or on the arm rests. Other times this can be getting her comfortable in bed with her feet propped on pillows. Whatever helps keep her comfortable and relaxed

Contractions: First, learn what Braxton Hicks contractions are and learn that they are not just 'fake' or something to 'blow off'. They hurt. A lot. These are basically practice contractions as delivery time gets closer. They can go anywhere from 30 seconds up to 2 minutes. But you need to learn the difference between these and real contractions that do-not-pass-go-and-head-to-the-hospital-now. If you aren't sure, research on the web or ask her doctor what to look for.

Easy dad recipes to make:

Getting tired of fast food? Here are more easy recipes!

Candied bacon little smokies: You'll need 2 packages of bacon (again I prefer precooked) cut into halves, 1 package of little smokies (any flavor you like), brown sugar, water, and toothpicks if you prefer them to hold pieces together. Preheat your oven to 350 and coat a baking dish with nonstick spray. In a medium bowl carefully stir together 1 cup of brown sugar and add in water in small amounts until the mix is a watery paste. Set that aside for now. Wrap the little smokies in a piece of bacon and place in the baking dish. I pack the little smokies together pretty tight so they are all coated evenly – if you use precooked bacon it's easier so you don't have to worry about the bacon being raw in places. Once you have all of the little smokies placed in the dish, carefully spoon all of the brown sugar mix evenly over all of the meat. Pop the dish in the oven and let it cook for about 12-15 minutes. The result: amazing melt in your mouth bacony goodness!

Turkey club cups: You'll need 12 slices of roasted turkey, 12 slices of sliced cheddar cheese, ¼ cup mayo, ½ head of iceberg lettuce (or whatever lettuce you prefer), 1 pint of cherry tomatoes, 8 slices of bacon cooked and chopped and a muffin tin. Start by preheating your oven to 400 degrees and spraying your muffin pan with cooking spray. Put a slice of turkey into each muffin cup then add a slice of cheddar. Pop that in the oven and bake until the turkey and cheese are pretty sturdy. Let them cool a bit and then spread a bit of the mayo in each cup. Add in lettuce, cherry tomatoes and bacon. You now have a great tasting easy meal (or snack)!

Zucchini sushi: (Don't worry, no raw fish involved!) You'll need 2 medium zucchini, 4 oz of cream cheese softened (just place in the microwave for a few seconds), 1 teaspoon of sriracha (if you want), 1 teaspoon lime juice, 1 cup of lump crab meat (yes, you can use the packaged fake stuff if you'd like, it tastes great too), ½ of a carrot cut into matchstick sizes, ½ avocado diced, ½ cucumber cut into matchstick sizes and 1 teaspoon toasted sesame seeds. Use a vegetable peeler and slice each zucchini into flat, thin strips. Peel the zucchini all the way down to the center. Place the strips on a paper towel lined plate or baking sheet. In a bowl, mix the sriracha, cream cheese and lime juice. Mix until it's smooth. Then lay the zucchini sliced out horizontally (long side facing you) and put a thin layer of the cream cheese mix on each one. Top the left side with a small bit of crab meat, carrots and cucumbers. Starting from that left side, carefully and tightly roll each zucchini slice. Then sprinkle with sesame seeds.

Chapter 7: The Third Trimester

The seventh month:

You guys are in the home stretch now. By about the 28th week, she's officially entered the third trimester and this is the last one before delivery. In fact, if you could peek inside, you would see pretty close to what it will look like when its born. The little peanut is the size of a large squash and can do a ton of things now, such as: blinking, coughing, hiccupping, reacting to sounds and touch and possibly even dreaming – wouldn't it be cool to know what they would have to dream about?

What's up with your partner:

This is the point when she will start having visits to the OBGYN every other week. Yes, this gets tiring, but it has to happen to ensure that any possible problems can be caught now. If the doctor has said that baby is in the wrong position, don't let her worry too much, you'd be surprised how quickly babies can flip flop in the womb.

Speaking of flip flopping, since her belly is growing and

baby is just growing like crazy too, her center of gravity will shift and it will make her a bit awkward with normal movements and walking. Help her sit or stand and make sure that she doesn't fall going up or down stairs or other areas where navigation may be harder. Her feet will also be expanding as her joints loosen to get ready for delivery. So, make sure that she's got comfortable shoes that she likes and that don't require tying or buckles. Comfy slip-ons are wonderful.

Since baby is now getting so big and has less room, it is going to mean her insides are getting more cramped, kicked, and resituated. She will be uncomfortable. She will be cranky. Just do what you can to help. Elbows, knees, legs, feet, hands and even that tiny head can get cramped up and just need to stretch. Now that the baby's bones are getting stronger, these movements will begin to be less exciting and more painful.

She also needs to make sure that she's getting at least 30mg of iron a day so anemia isn't a problem after the baby is born. Of course, this also means that it will make her constipated which in turn causes less room in that already cramped space. Write down a reminder for her to ask the doctor what she can do to help this problem. Just don't blurt it out at the doctor for her.

What's up with the peanut:

While kiddo may look pretty close to who you'll meet in a few weeks, it's little organs still have some growing to do. Its brain is learning to make faster connections for higher thinking powers as well as normal bodily functions that it will need to survive.

Speaking of the brain, now is the time that peanut's brain really kicks into gear. More wrinkles are developing in the brain as more nerve cell connections are established. As the brain matures, the baby's senses will grow as well. You'll notice that it is more aware of light, sound and touch. One of our favorite things to do was lightly push in one area and get a response – either right under your fingers or on the other side of the belly. It's almost like a game you can play before birth.

At this point, the little peanut will have settled into a schedule with being asleep and awake. Of course, I'm warning you now, this won't always coincide with your schedules. Don't be alarmed if you're woken by a kick in the middle of the night.

What's up with you:

At this point, she will also be putting on about a pound or so per week because baby is plumping up also. While I don't recommend getting between a pregnant woman and the food's she is craving, I do recommend keeping different vitamins and other great pregnancy foods around to make sure that deficiencies aren't an issue.

Along with her putting on some weight, you'll probably notice that you are as well. Chances are that you're eating what she is, which means weird cravings – sitting up at 3 am eating broccoli and cheese, pancakes at 3 in the afternoon, running to some obscure restaurant across town because she wants their specific type of queso… there's really no way that you aren't going to gain a bit. However, here's my advice: don't go overboard with griping about it or making sure that she notices you're working out more. This isn't going to help her any and will probably mean you're going to bear the brunt of a lot of fights. Sure, it's upsetting to gain a bit of weight, but remember that she has no choice in gaining some weight with the baby and you don't want to do or say anything that will make her feel bad for having a baby.

Key things to do this month:

Other people's comments: While 99% of things people say to a pregnant woman are positive, there will be that one time when someone makes a rude comment. Whether it's someone at the mall saying she's just really fat or your mother talking about how much weight she's gained (I've had both of these happen personally and you don't want her to hear this, trust me), it will happen. The best thing that you can do is to immediately stop anyone saying something within her earshot – family especially. Remind them that she's pregnant. She's carrying your child. And that all you care about is a healthy baby and a healthy happy mommy. When it comes to other people's comments, learn the fine art of being a smartass that will make them feel about an inch tall. During our shopping trip to the mall, a lady and her teenage daughter were eating at a couple of tables down from us. For some reason, it was fun for them to snicker and make fat comments when my wife got up to get a drink or throw something away. My wife never heard them and I never told her. When we went to leave, I made sure to walk behind my wife and lean over and whisper 'She's carrying twins. Thank you for pointing out how wonderful she looks.' Both of them looked horrified, the mother quickly began to repeat how sorry she was but it was fun just to walk away with my beautiful wife.

Hospital extras: Since you have been hitting the doctor's office with her, you should already have a plan of what hospital you're heading to. I highly recommend that you go up to the hospital and just drive around, find out where to park by the entrance that you need to head into, where exits are for the parking lots, easiest areas to park in and all of those little things that you won't think of until you're stressed out trying to get her to the hospital.

Nice things to do for your partner this month:

Snack bags: I learned that my wife got hungry for snacky items when we weren't anywhere near a restaurant or home. So, I began to pack little snack bags for her with some of her favorite treats. Yes, I tried to include some healthy snacks too, however it's hard to deny a pregnant woman her cravings. Granola bars, trail mix, and other small items like this can easily fit into small zip lock bags that you can slide into her purse, the glovebox, etc. She'll love you for it.

Shopping: Yes, yes, you've been shopping more than you wanted for baby stuff. However, this is for her.

Take her out and let her pick out some loose fitting clothes to wear home from the hospital as well as comfy pajamas and a robe. Don't just try to find something, you'll end up with something she hates. Instead, take her out and take some time just for you two. Go to lunch and then walk around the mall. Walk around the baby isles and baby megastores, looking at items. Just enjoy some time alone.

Easy dad recipes to make:

Here are more easy recipes that you can tackle when she's not feeling up to cooking or you want to be nice:

Easy awesome baked potatoes: While you can bake potatoes in the oven, I prefer the easier route and hit the microwave. Usually about 10 minutes on high will do a medium sized potato. So, here are two different routes for easy potatoes:

1. Oven: Preheat the oven to about 350. Wash off the potatoes, slice them down the middle and take out a little frustration stabbing them in different places to allow steam to get out and the meat to cook better. I put a spoonful of butter down the middle of my potatoes and salt and pepper. Wrap each potato in foil and place on a baking sheet. Place in the oven for about 20-30 minutes, checking about every 10

minutes to see how soft they are.

2. Microwave: Wash the potatoes and slice and stab as directed above. Put that spoonful of butter and salt and pepper down the middle. DO NOT wrap them in foil for the microwave. You don't want that fire and sparking light show. Place potatoes on a microwave safe plate and cook for 10 minutes. Check to make sure that they are done to your liking, putting them back in for extra time if needed.

While potatoes are cooking, I usually make some broccoli, chop up roast beef, tomatoes, cheese and really any other toppings that you can think of. There are some crazy ways to dress up a potato and you can do something different every single night if you want. My personal favorites are bacon, broccoli and cheese and chopped barbecue brisket.

Banana split pops: Ok, so this one is more of a desert, but it is easy and great, especially in the hot summer months. You'll need 4 bananas, 8 popsicle sticks, 1 cup melted chocolate (usually you can find chocolate dip in the fruit section of your local grocery store, just heat it, dip and put back in the freezer), ½ cup sprinkles, whipped cream and cherries. Line a baking sheet with wax paper and set aside. Cut the ends off the bananas and then cut in half. Put a popsicle stick into each banana, place it on the baking sheet and freeze for 2 hours. After those 2 hours, heat up the chocolate and put in a dipping bowl if it doesn't already come in one. Pour sprinkles into a bowl. Then dip each banana into the chocolate and roll it in the sprinkles. Place back on baking sheet and put back into freezer when they are all coated. After about 30 minutes, you can take them out of the freezer to serve, just add whipped cream and a cherry to the top!

Chicken bacon ranch wraps: You'll need 2 boneless chicken breasts OR deli sliced chicken, salt, pepper, 2 roma tomatoes sliced thin, romaine lettuce (leaf form works best, but you can easily use the salad mix type at the grocery store), tortillas (although you can use the large romaine leaves as the wrap instead if you'd like), provolone or whatever sliced cheese you'd like), 8-10 strips of cooked bacon and ranch. If you go with chicken breasts, make sure that you cook them or that you buy precooked ones. On a baking sheet or cutting board lay out paper towels, wax paper, parchment or any other type of cooking paper you'd like, lay out the tortilla or the large romaine leaf. Then line each one with 2 slices of cheese on the bottom, then tomatoes, then bacon, then chicken. Put ranch on the top and sprinkle with salt and pepper to your liking. Tightly wrap the leaf or tortilla around the mix and use a toothpick to hold it closed. Serve and enjoy!

Chapter 8: Home Stretch

The eighth month:

Some days it will seem like you'll never get everything done before the baby arrives and other days it will seem like forever until it's time to meet the little kiddo. Baby starts out the eighth month about the size of a large cantaloupe and will enter the ninth month about the size of a large honeydew melon or a small seedless watermelon. (I'm getting hungry for fruit, how about you?)

What's up with your partner:

Even though there is less room for baby to wiggle around, the wiggling will continue. Sometimes this will mean that baby will stretch out in a weird position and she'll be struggling to move or even take a good breath (yes, baby can stretch so far that it can push up against her lungs). If you see that she is really uncomfortable, ask what you can do to help. Sometimes having someone else involved can ease that worry that these stretches can bring – especially when they don't go away very fast.

Along with the wonderful movements of that little kiddo and the fun of baby showers and attention, there are some ugly sides to pregnancy during this month. We've already talked about heartburn and how bad it can get. Well, as baby gets bigger, this gets worse. Keep stashes of antacids in the car, bags, drawers, bedside, bathroom and really any other place that you can think of. Along with this issue, hemorrhoids are a common, and painful, reality to being pregnant. If these issues are bothersome (and face it, when would they not be), mention that she should ask her doctor about them. Write it down in the notebook if you need to, but don't make a big issue out of it. Chances are that she's pretty embarrassed about the whole situation already.

Sleep is a commodity that she cannot get enough of during these last months. Baby stays asleep and calm while she's moving since it's a constant rocking rhythm. When she lays down to rest, well that's a whole different ball game. Usually when she's trying to rest, baby wakes up because there is no movement. So, hey, it's time to play! With little sleep at night, chances are that she'll be needing naps throughout the day. If you do find that she's fallen asleep on the couch, the recliner or in bed, make sure that she is comfortable (without waking her, such as covering her with a blanket and so on) and then keeping everything quiet so she can nap.

She will start to notice that baby is sitting further down in her pelvis and chances are that she'll feel it exactly when this happens. Some doctors will call this 'lightening' others will say 'the baby has dropped', no matter which one they call it, it just means that baby is getting ready for delivery. The good side: she'll be able to breathe easier. The bad side: it means more trips to the bathroom as now baby is sitting on her bladder.

WHAT'S UP WITH THE PEANUT:

You already know that little peanut has been growing like crazy, but now is when things really start to develop and give personality to your kiddo. That fine body hair called lanugo is falling off and little kiddo only has hair on its head, eyebrows and eyelashes now.

As the month goes on, baby's bones will begin to finally harden to support it outside of the womb. The only bone that won't do this is your baby's skull. It still needs to be pliable to fit through the birth canal, and a soft spot will remain on the top of kiddo's noggin for a while after birth. Make sure that you understand what this is and how to protect it.

During this month, baby's organs will grow and develop so that they will be able to work on their own very soon.

Baby will shift into the head-down position, but if this doesn't happen, don't worry. Sometimes babies wait until the last minute to shift, sometimes they have to be manually shifted by the doctor and other times, it's just C-section time. (No matter which way your kiddo decides to make its entrance, the doctor will be ready.)

What's up with you:

I know that I've already mentioned anxiety and nerves, but they will really start to blow up when you realize that you're a month or less away from having a newborn in the house. One thing that has helped me is to ensure the house is secure, either with an alarm system or monitors on the windows and doors (you don't need expensive ones, you can easily pick up the lower priced ones that attach on the window or door and the frame). These monitors will go off if the window or door opens.

You can also read up on what to expect at the hospital, terminology that you aren't familiar with, newborn care and other items that you aren't sure about. There really is no such thing as learning too much.

Key things to do this month:

DHA rich foods: DHA is an essential nutrient for growing babies' brains. You'll start to notice that DHA is in all sorts of formulas and baby foods, but baby needs it now too. One of the best ways to get this is fish like salmon that are rich in DHA. There are supplements too, but they aren't as fun to take since they can look like horse pills. Plus, if she's craving fish, you can find several types that will offer great amounts of DHA. (Just make sure that you're paying attention to the levels of mercury in some farm raised fish.)

When the water breaks: Everyone has heard horror stories and seen movies where the woman's water breaks at the worst time possible. While this doesn't happen a lot, it can happen when you aren't ready. So be ready. Know what this means and what you need to do when it happens. If you aren't sure about the information that you're reading online (because we all know that every different site will say something else), ask her doctor. Make sure that you have a good understanding of what to do so you can be calm when she isn't.

Episiotomies and you: Not many men know what this means, I sure didn't. When I did find out, I wish I didn't know. However, it's part of birth. An episiotomy is a surgical cut in the muscle between the vagina and the anus before delivery to give the baby more room. These used to be extremely common and are starting to become something that's bypassed now. However, you should know what it is just in case.

Baby position: When you're at the doctor, make sure that you both are getting updates on the baby's position and what that means for delivery. The doctor will be monitoring this every time she visits, so write down questions, concerns or comments to mention when you guys are at your next visit. You don't want any surprises when you head to the delivery room with the doctor saying 'I told you this already'.

Nice things to do for your partner this month:

Telling people 'no': When you're pregnant, everyone wants to touch your belly. Some women don't care and love people feeling the baby kick. Others won't want just anyone putting their hands on their belly. Talk to your partner about this and discuss what to say and do if she's uncomfortable with having someone touch her. Also, make sure that you're ready to stand up and say 'no' if she is too shy or worried about offending someone. Be the bad guy here, it's ok.

Easy dad recipes to make:

More easy recipes for you to please your partner and others:

BLT cups: You'll need 12-15 slices of uncooked bacon, either bacon bits or other cooked bacon chopped up, 2 teaspoons of lemon juice (if you like), salt, black pepper, 2 cups of cherry tomatoes cut in halves, 1 chopped head of lettuce (or you can cheat like I do and buy the precut stuff at the grocery store), shredded cheese of your choice and any other toppings that you'd like. Preheat your oven to 400 and invert your muffin pan to have large upside down cups. Cut 8 slices of the bacon in half and cover the upside down cups. Wrap the outsides of that layer of bacon so that it will form an entire bacon cup when cooked. Bake until the bacon is crispy and solid, but don't burn it. Let the bacon cups cool for about 15 minutes or so. Carefully remove the bacon cups when they are cooled off and fill them with lettuce, tomato and more bacon. Add shredded cheese, salt and pepper to taste.

Pepperoni pizza swirls: You'll need a large ball of pizza dough OR the premade packaged dough that already comes in a sheet (you can use the ones in the spaghetti/pizza sauce isle or you can use the Pillsbury canned dough, both are great), ¼ cup marinara sauce, 8 oz of sliced mozzarella and 8 oz of pepperoni. Preheat your oven to 400 and line a baking sheet with foil. Roll out the dough into a long rectangle. Spread a thin layer of sauce leaving about a little over a ½ inch clear around the border on the sides. Evenly layer the pepperonis and then cover with an even layer of cheese. Then tightly and carefully roll the dough up into a long jelly roll. Carefully transfer to the baking sheet if you didn't roll it there to begin with – you want the seam side down on the baking sheet. Cook for about 10-15 minutes (depending on your oven). Let cool for 5 minutes, slice into ½ to 1 inch slices and serve!

Melting pigs in a blanket: You'll need sliced cheese (we use the Kraft slices because they melt better), hot dogs or little smokies, melted butter, Pillsbury crescent roll dough OR regular canned biscuits and salt. Preheat your oven to 350 and spray a baking sheet or cover in foil. If using hot dogs, cut them in half. Then do the following depending on your dough choice:

1. Crescent roll dough already comes in triangles so it's easier to use. Roll out the dough and separate the triangles. Starting at the thick end, put a slide of cheese and a hot dog or smokie down on top of the cheese. Carefully, and not too tightly, roll the dough toward the small end. Place on the baking sheet. Repeat for the

rest of the dough. Brush the melted butter over the tops and sprinkle with salt.

2. Open the biscuits and lay them out on a baking sheet. Start by spreading out one biscuit with your fingers until it's about twice the size it was. Place a slice of cheese and a hot dog or smokie in the middle and roll the sides together. Place on the baking sheet with the seam side down. Brush with butter and add salt.

Place in the oven for about 12 minutes, or until the tops are golden brown. Serve and enjoy.

Chapter 9: Here Comes Baby

The ninth month:

There is absolutely no way to gauge how long labor will take so neither one of you should try. Generally, labor can last anywhere from 12 to 36 hours when someone is having their first baby, but don't bet the farm on that either. Just remember when she says she needs to go to the hospital, don't wait around to watch the last 20 minutes of that basketball game. Go. Now. Chances are good that she will have to be in the early phase of labor for several hours before the hospital will even admit her. If you can, spend time together and help to keep her from worrying. Once it's time to go to the hospital again, go calmly, don't freak out.

You also need to realize that labor is extremely painful and no, you have never and will never understand. There are pain measures that the doctor will take to help her but it will still be beyond painful. It may seem like nothing is happening to you, but she is still having contractions and other symptoms the whole time. Focus on helping her feel comfortable, such as getting ice chips, giving foot rubs, back rubs or cold washcloths. Anything you can to for her will be greatly appreciated.

There will be times during labor that she will tell you to get the hell out of the delivery room. Never, I repeat: NEVER, walk out. Stay right where you are and ignore the mean spew that can come out of her mouth. She's in extreme pain, keep that in mind.

What's up with your partner:

Pregnancy brain fog is a real and frustrating part of pregnancy and it will happen. She will get frustrated and upset, so do not yell or get mad at her for forgetting something. If it is really bad, offer to help write things down or set reminders on her phone. The hormones that go along with pregnancy will be causing crazy things to happen and she'll be getting less than great sleep for a long time. Combine both of those and you have a recipe for forgetting everything. Just remember that this type of brain fog is common and it will pass.

Your partner will feel like she's carrying around a bowling ball and it will start to seem that way. Her back is going to start taking on more strain as delivery gets closer. Keep this in mind when you feel that her back can't possibly be hurting that much. It does. And it will continue to for a while even after the baby is born.

The baby weighs anywhere from 6 to 9 pounds during this last month, and sometimes more. So, all of that extra weight right in the front will also pull her stomach muscles as well as strain her legs. Do everything you can to help you get around.

What's up with the peanut:

The baby is now full term, even at 36 weeks. Kiddo will be getting ready to make its appearance by moving its head down further into her pelvis. Your baby's immune system is also taking on information from the mother's body. All of the organs are fully functional and ready to go. Baby's brain is beginning to control its body instead of relying on the mother's body.

What's up with you:

No matter how anxious you may feel about labor and the birth, try to hide that from her as best as possible. She will be a million times more worried than you are and her brain will be working nonstop. Do your best to reassure her everything will go smoothly and the baby will be perfect. If you pile any fears or worries on her, they will only multiply her own feelings.

You may also be worried about contractions and what do to. Hopefully you've taken my advice and learned the difference between real contractions and Braxton Hicks. If not, shame on you (just kidding). Do so now. Also you should know what point you should head to the hospital when contractions are regular and a certain interval appart.

Key things to do this month:

Pack those bags early: You will need a bag for baby, one for her and one for you. Plan on staying two nights in the hospital (even though usually it will be just one for normal deliveries). Have extra items to wear with you both as newborns can be messy. There is a list at the end of this book to help you with what you guys need and what baby needs.

Nursery time: You probably already have this finished, but you want to help her with getting the nursery around before baby comes home. Put together furniture, sort out baby items, put things where they need to go, stock up the changing table… and, well, you get the idea. Basically, be almost over prepared before you head to the hospital.

Nice things to do for your partner this month:

Stress relief: I guarantee that she is stressing out severely under that excitement. Take the time to do things to help her relax. This can include massage, foot rubs, relaxing bubble baths, scented candles she loves, swimming or other activities that she enjoys. Help keep her mind off of the terrible things that are floating around in her head. If she begins to bring up 'what if' questions, remind her that her doctor is experienced and great in this area and she's in good hands.

Nesting: All pregnant women go through a phase toward the end of the pregnancy called 'nesting'. She may be going through baby clothes and nursery items repeatedly, moving, rearranging, and making sure everything is 'perfect' to her. She'll also do this around the house as well and feel like there won't be enough time to get everything perfect before baby arrives. Here is what you should do: help. Even if she's moved the nursery around seven times, move it again. Chances are that you'll end up with things in the same places that you started from, but just smile and do it. It will help her feel better and less cramped for time.

Easy dad recipes to make:

Pigs in a quilt: You'll need 1 tube of the Pillsbury French bread dough, 6-8 hot dogs, melted butter and salt. Preheat your oven to 375. Roll out dough into a large rectangle then cut into 8 thin strips. Here's the part that you can decide what you do: you can either lay the strips down and alternate flipping the strips up to weave in the hot dogs OR you can put the hotdogs down and lay the strips over them, poking the areas between the hot dogs down. Once you've got that part done, brush the melted butter over the tops of the dough and sprinkle with salt. Pop in the oven for about 20 minutes until the dough is golden brown. Cut and serve with any dips you want.

Fish stick tacos: You'll need 1 package of premade fish sticks, salt, pepper, tortillas, chopped salad mix of your choosing, shredded cheddar cheese, chopped tomatoes and salsa if you'd like. First, cook the fish sticks following the directions on the box or bag. Then lay out the tortillas and place 2-4 fish sticks down the middle (more or less if you'd like), then top with the lettuce mix, cheese, tomatoes, salt and pepper. Add salsa or put in a bowl for dipping. Serve and enjoy!

Easy Frito pie: You'll need 1 bag of Fritos, 1 can of premade chili, shredded cheese and jalapenos, onions or other toppings you like. Heat the chili up according to the directions. Put a layer of Fritos in a bowl, then top with a layer of chili, then add layer of shredded cheese. You can either top with another small layer of Fritos or other toppings that you'd like. Mmmmm... Frito chili pie!

The Baby is Finally Here!

It's finally over – now what? Baby is here and you're overwhelmed with all of the things that go into taking care of a newborn. Don't worry though, people have been doing it for centuries and will continue to do so for a very long time.

What's up with your partner:

She will suddenly be super worried about losing baby weight. Reassure her so she doesn't stress and stop eating. However, steer clear of gyms and other 'gift' items for weight loss. If she mentions it, then you can slowly agree. Don't jump on the chance because you will say something that offends her. I'm mentioning this first because I made this mistake with our first child and I'm trying to spare others the evil dagger eyes and the comments about your own weight, where you can stick your comments and general miserable times afterward… for a long time. She won't forget, believe me.

She also will be doting on that tiny human you just brought home from the hospital. Remember that she is the one doing the majority of the work and still probably still exhausted and sore from delivery. Help wherever you can. She loves that little human, but she still needs to take time for herself. Just a hot shower and clean clothes can make all the difference if she's having a hard day. Offer to let her nap while you take care of the baby. Order her favorite meal and pick it up for her.

Some women also develop post-partum depression and there is treatment that her doctor can provide to help if this happens. You should learn the signs and what to do if you see any symptoms of post-partum depression. If it's something you are worried about, call her doctor or doctor's nurse and talk with them. They can help with evaluating and treatment if necessary. However, don't just assume that she has post-partum depression if she's tired or cranky. There are true symptoms that will stand out from her normal routine and self.

What's up with the peanut:

Baby weighs anywhere between 6 to 10 pounds at this point at is about 20 inches long. Kiddo sleeps a lot, eats a lot and goes through diapers a lot. But it is a perfect little human that you brought into the world. Enjoy all of those times when the eyes are open and fixed on you. Take too many pictures. Video everything. Keep everything. These first few days and couple of weeks are quiet times that you can just stare and awe at this tiny baby. After the first month or so, things will start to pick up and before you know it, there will be first bites of food, first sounds, first words, first rolling over, first pushing up on its arms, first crawls, first steps and the list goes on. So, enjoy these first couple of weeks and the beautiful little thing as it sleeps in your arms.

Your baby will sleep… and sleep… and sleep. When you first come home, chances are that kiddo will sleep up to 16 hours a day – just not all at one time. Some babies will sleep through the night a few days after coming home and others you'll be fighting to get out of your bed and sleep all night when they are four. Every kid is different. If you are woke up during the night with baby cries, wait just a moment to see if baby goes back to sleep. If not, quietly go in, change diapers, feed, whatever you need to do, but do it quietly and calmly. If not, you're going to wake kiddo up more and you won't be headed back to bed any time soon.

Actively talk and interact with the baby during the day. Doing this will help ensure that baby is awake during the day and sleeps at night.

Infants will eat about every 2 to 3 hours for those eating formula and about 1 to 2 hours if breastfeeding. Of course, again, every baby is different. If you notice that baby is going too long between feedings or doesn't want to eat, talk to the pediatrician. If baby is eating formula, you may try a different brand. With our second child, breastfeeding wasn't working and then we went through four types of formula before we found on that worked. It happens. It's not the end of the world I promise.

Baths during the first month or so should be limited to 3 or less a week. If you do it more, you can dry out that soft new skin. You do want to make sure that you wait until the umbilical cord has fallen off and healed a bit before that first bath.

Keeping baby's bottom dry and clean is key. Nothing is worse than a kiddo with diaper rash. It's painful and baby won't be able to sleep or be comfortable at all. Changing diapers often will help keep any pee or poop from staying on the skin too long. Remember that newborns have very sensitive skin so be gentle when cleaning the areas. Don't use textured wipes and pat the area dry with a soft towel. It's also a good idea to use wipes that do NOT have fragrances or alcohol in them. These can irritate the skin and cause problems.

You also need to make sure that you aren't putting on diapers too tight as that can also cut off some circulation in baby's legs and just make them uncomfortable.

What's up with you:

You're excited that baby is here but nervous at the same time. Don't worry, you're not going to drop your newborn. Trust me. You'll hold on to that tiny thing like your life depended on it. As you hold the baby more and you're used to carrying the peanut around, you'll get more comfortable and that fear will go away.

Oh diapers. Let's talk about diapers. You probably had already decided that you'd never change a diaper, that you'd throw up if you saw or smelled poo. But you won't. You want to jump in and help with diapers period. Don't just leave all of that to her because she's the woman. If you let her do it all, that means she's up throughout the night with feedings and diapers too. It also means that she has no break at all from baby. Yes, she will need breaks. Everyone gets worn out sometimes and you should try to give her time to relax and just take a breath.

I already mentioned this above, but I'm going to say it again: help. Don't be one of those dads that believes she should do everything from feeding to diapers to rocking... you get the point. Just help.

Key things to do now:

Post-delivery C-section care: If she had a C-section, she will need more help than if she had a normal birth. So, make sure that you listened carefully to the doctor's instructions and wrote things down that you didn't want to forget. Trust me, she will be pretty on the ball with what she needs to do to care for herself, but there will be times when she'll forget. Remember that she had her stomach muscle walls sliced open for a C-section and these will take a while to heal and work properly. Her back will also be sore and she may still have some after effects from the anesthesia. If you have to go back to work in a couple of days, I recommend getting someone to come stay with her while you're not home. Family and friends are usually happy to help so they can snuggle that tiny human. C-sections are harder on a woman than a natural birth, but everything will go back to normal as long as you help her remember to take care of herself.

Post-delivery natural birth care: If she had a natural birth, there isn't as much to worry about with surgery incisions and so on. However, she will still be really sore and need help those first two weeks or so. Just like with a C-section, if you have to go back to work soon, have someone come stay with her. It will make both of you feel better and provide company for her.

Bond with baby: Bonding is one of the most rewarding

things that you can possibly do. And, guess what, it's not hard! Hold your infant close to you and make sure that you have some areas of skin touching, arms, that tiny head on your chest, etc. You also should talk to the baby, sing, whisper, read – anything that gives baby more time to hear your voice and get to know you. Eye contact and smiles are also a great way to bond. Even if baby doesn't smile back right away, it won't take long until peanut is mimicking you.

Nice things to do for your partner:

Gifts: I recommend bringing her a gift to commemorate the baby's birth. This can be anything from a mother's ring or necklace to something like a framed photo of the baby's first picture. Name a star after the baby or after her (yes, I know it's just 'fake' or 'pretend' but she will love it) and frame the certificate. Just any thing that is personal that you can do to show her you love her more than she'll ever know. You don't have to go overboard – unless you want to – but just do things that will make her feel special.

Visiting schedules: No, you're not running a prison here but you should make schedules for when to have people over and when it's time for you and her and baby. Don't be forceful about it, but do make sure that you let people know you have planned baby time together at a certain time. People will understand and will be happy to let you have your time. If you have a relative or friend that is really pushy, don't get rude or hateful. Just make sure that they know you expect them to let you have time alone and if necessary form a plan to get everyone out to have some peace and quiet.

Easy dad recipes to make:

Ok, I'm not going to fib here. Chances are that people will be bringing over food after you guys are home from the hospital. If not, or you just hate what they are bringing, I suggest that you stock up on quick fix frozen meals. There are complete meals, corn dogs, chicken strips, fish planks and so much more in your freezer isle at the grocery store. This way, you can throw something in the oven, grab it when it's done and not have to worry about standing in the kitchen cooking. I mean, hey, you've got that beautiful little kiddo to snuggle!

If people are bringing stuff over that you don't like, don't tell them so. They went out of their way to bring over food to help you guys out. Instead, politely accept the dish and put it in the fridge or wherever it needs to go and eat something else later.

Helpful Tips and Information

Here at the end, I wanted to include some tips, checklists and other information that you will need to know during and after the pregnancy. Hopefully these will help you out, I didn't have a lot of this information during our first pregnancy and I sure wish I had.

Hospital Bag Checklist:

These are the items that you want to have packed and ready before you ever think it is time to head to the hospital:

Grown up list:

- ✓ Loose fitting, comfy clothing for her to wear home
- ✓ Something for you to wear home
- ✓ Toiletries – toothbrushes, floss, etc
- ✓ Insurance information and any hospital forms
- ✓ Birth plan (if you have one)
- ✓ Family phone numbers to call when baby is here
- ✓ Warm, nonskid socks for her
- ✓ Warm robe that you don't mind throwing away later
- ✓ Maternity bras – NO underwire, she'll thank you, trust me
- ✓ Lip balm
- ✓ Headbands and pony tail holders if she has long hair
- ✓ Hard candy to help during labor when she can't eat
- ✓ Pen and paper
- ✓ Change for the vending machines
- ✓ Cell phone chargers

- ✓ Camera (if you want, most people use their phones)

Baby and diaper bag list:
- ✓ CAR SEAT!!!! They won't allow you to leave the hospital with the baby if you don't have a car seat
- ✓ Diapers
- ✓ Wipes
- ✓ Hand sanitizer
- ✓ Changing pad
- ✓ Plastic or disposable bags
- ✓ Bottles and formula if she isn't breastfeeding
- ✓ Extra soft baby blankets
- ✓ Clothing for the baby – you want to have a few outfits for mishaps
- ✓ Pacifier
- ✓ Nursing cover if she's breastfeeding

Of course, there will be special things that you'll want to include in both your bag and baby's bag. Just make sure that you have them ready to go before you actually need to walk out the door.

Items to Include in a Birth Plan:

I mentioned a birth plan in the previous chapters so I thought I would list a few of the different things that are normally included in one:

1. Insurance information
2. Delivery doctor
3. Pediatrician
4. What type of child birth she would like: natural, no drugs, epidural, etc
5. Do you want photos or videos in the delivery room (if permitted)
6. Who does she want in the delivery room
7. Is there anyone that you don't want in the delivery room
8. Does she want to stand up, use a shower, walk around or lie down during labor
9. Is there a birthing position she would prefer
10. Does she want fetal monitoring (normally this is done no matter what, but some hospitals give the choice)
11. Does she have feelings either way about assisted deliveries – this includes vacuum extractions and forceps
12. If she has to have a C-section, does she want you in the room
13. Does she want to cut the umbilical cord or let you

14. Does she want to hold the baby right away or wait until it's washed off – if she has a C-section, they may not allow her to hold the baby right away until her medications wear off
15. If you're having a boy, do you both want him circumcised

There may be other items that she will want on her birth plan. Help her look at different options as well as items that she may not consider.

Great Foods During Pregnancy:

Here is a short list of foods that are excellent for her to chomp on while she's pregnant:

1. Breakfast cereal fortified with B vitamins and other vitamins and supplements
2. Dried beans and lentils for protein
3. Salmon for omega-3 fatty acids and DHA
4. Broccoli offers calcium, fiber and antioxidants
5. Nonfat milk for calcium
6. Sweet potatoes for vitamin A, vitamin C, fiber and folate
7. Bananas for potassium, nausea, energy and to fight off leg cramps
8. Lean meat for protein and iron
9. Cheeses for calcium and protein
10. Colorful fruits and veggies for fiber, minerals and giving the baby the ability to love these foods later on
11. Walnuts for omega-3s, proteins and DHA
12. Eggs for protein and amino acids
13. Oatmeal for energy, carbs, and lowering cholesterol
14. Leafy greens for iron, fiber, protein, folate and vitamins A, C and K
15. Greek yogurt for calcium and probiotics
16. Whole grain breads for fiber
17. Oranges for vitamin C, fiber, folate and water

18. Dried fruits for vitamins and to curb sugar cravings
19. Avocado for vitamins and nutrients
20. Lots of water to keep her hydrated

You can also ask the doctor if there are any foods that she can recommend or if there are other supplements on top of prenatal vitamins that she should take.

Realistic Dad Information:

There are always things that you assume will go one way – and then they end up blowing up in your face. Here are some hard realizations that you'll want to understand right away:

1. As soon as you guys announce that she's pregnant – be prepared for her to be the center of attention... the whole time. Be mentally prepared and don't get upset. It's nothing personal.
2. When baby gets here, she will still be getting most of the attention, but the clear majority of attention will be on that little peanut.
3. If you're making either set of your parent's grandparents for the first time, give them a bit to soak that in. They may be ecstatic about the baby, but there will be that shock that they are becoming grandparents.
4. Hormones will make it seem like she suddenly has multiple personalities. Just learn to deal with them and be nice.
5. For the first two to three weeks, being pregnant will be amazing. After the genetic testing, amniocentesis, information on breech births and C-sections, lectures about what can go wrong during birth, maxing your credit cards on baby stuff and so on – you'll develop a mix

of elation and anxiety for your child forever. You should hug your parents as you now know what they've been through with you.

6. Suddenly your house will become too small. She will remind you of this all the time. Don't worry about it and don't argue. Just say "I know" and whatever else you can to make her feel better – without promising a new house.

7. When baby gets here – and well before – you'll be broke. Seriously. Don't consider buying new clothes, TVs, man toys, etc. You won't have time to appreciate them right now anyway. Plus, there will always be money for baby items, such as multiple car seats, cribs, strollers, tons of clothes, diapers, toys and the list goes on.

8. However, go out and buy new tires for the cars now. That will be one of the larger things that can easily go wrong trying to get her to the hospital when the baby's coming. Trust me on this.

9. Lamaze sounds like a waste of time... until you're in the delivery room and have no idea what to do. Just suck it up and go.

10. Get used to her changing her birth plan and her mind about labor repeatedly. She'll want a midwife. She'll want a birthing center. She'll want two doctors. She'll want the pediatrician to be there when she gives birth. Then she will

only want one doctor. And she'll hate the pediatrician she picked out. She'll want to have a natural birth. Then she'll scream for that epidural. She'll want a cesarean. Then she won't. Just agree with her and move on. It will all work out in the end and it's not worth the arguments.
11. If she decides that she wants that epidural, don't ask if she's really sure. Just get the doctor because yes, she's sure.
12. The only time that screaming and pushing will ever make your relationship better is in the delivery room.
13. She will be able to out-smell 50 bloodhounds. Get used to it. Don't offer to take her to a search and rescue team.
14. Contractions are not funny and you cannot blow them off. Period. They also won't be the same as the little chart that you'll get at Lamaze classes. Ever. When she says it's time to go to the hospital – it's time to go to the hospital.
15. They will tell you that you're the coach – but you're really not. There will come a time during her labor that you'll just have to shush and watch. Let her finish that last touchdown. Then step in and cut the ribbon.
16. Be careful using the word 'we' when talking about the pregnancy or the birth. "We didn't mind amniocentesis", "We knew the C-section

wouldn't be that bad" and so on are no-nos. Just think before you use the word 'we'.

17. No matter how many movies you've seen this in: you won't faint. No one ever does in the real world.
18. Sex while pregnant will not hurt the baby. Also, 'sex' will not be 'sex' for at least a year or so. It will be 'making love'. Get used to it.
19. Suddenly she'll eat like a trucker on a long haul. Do not say a word. She's feeding your kid. Just smile and go buy that second birthday cake because she's craving it.
20. Also unlike movies, yes, you must be in the delivery room.
21. Do not give her a gym membership, a piece of workout equipment or anything revolving around her getting back into shape. It. Will. Backfire.
22. Don't overshare about being pregnant at work. You can do that when your home.
23. However, tell everyone and their dog about the birth. This is the time anyone and everyone will be truly ecstatic for you.
24. By the time you change that third diaper, you'll be a pro and nothing will surprise you.
25. There are things that you just knew would make you sick: baby pee, baby poop and baby puke. But they won't. And you'll get used to them all... usually because you'll be wearing

them all at once.
26. Your mom or her mom will pull you aside and tell you how breastfeeding will either ruin her breasts or make her lose weight faster, how babies only need to be fed every four hours or how you should just feel them constantly and how you need to let them 'cry it out' or how you should always go check. You'll figure it out and do it your own way.
27. After the kiddo is here, friends who have no children will suddenly have tons of advice for you. Friends with kids will simply smile and say "It'll pass. Don't worry." Listen to the ones with kids.
28. Memorize the following things: Boppy, Baby Bjorn, Gerber, My Breast Friend and other baby item names.
29. When baby gets here, you will be amazed at how well you function on such a small amount of sleep.
30. It's still an enigma on why babies need so many clothes. You won't figure it out either.
31. Yes, it's normal to stare at that sweet, sleeping baby face for hours.
32. It's normal to think every newborn baby smile is a smile. People will say 'it's just gas'. Always consider it a smile and be happy.
33. It's also normal to take tons of video and photos of your baby sleeping, in new clothes,

eating and just looking around.
34. During your second week home, you'll learn to love casseroles, lasagna and other weird dishes people bring over.
35. Yes, you will always be holding the baby wrong unless you do it her way.
36. You'll suddenly understand why all of your friends with newborns never want you to come visit and never want to come visit – unless you're bringing food over or offering a good dinner.
37. Breast milk is like spinach to Popeye. Don't insist on 50 pre-made bottles in the fridge.
38. You'll suddenly understand why there are dads at the stores who are dressed in sweats and a cotton shirt.
39. No matter what, your kiddo will always like Gerber foods better than anything you make from scratch. Plus, it's easier to buy Gerber than make it yourself. Don't listen to what anyone else says. After that first batch of homemade baby food, you'll be so done with it you'll buy stock in Gerber.
40. No, you can't trade in gifts for take-out or diapers.
41. You never realized how many diapers babies go through – or how expensive that becomes.
42. During that third month after the baby is born, you'll still have to love lasagna and casseroles.

43. The baby will like her better for a while. It's nothing personal. Your turn will come along.
44. Sometime after the baby arrives, she will want to go on a 'date'. Halfway through said date, you'll both start worrying about the baby and go home instead of seeing that movie.
45. Nannies aren't lactation consultants, day nurses aren't midwives and gynecologists aren't pediatricians. Learn what each one of those jobs entails.
46. After more family visiting your house than you've ever seen in 20 years, you'll suddenly appreciate "Everybody Loves Raymond".
47. No matter how frustrated you get with diapers, bottles, breast feeding, no sleep and sleeping by yourself because she's up rocking the baby – just take a breath and enjoy it. This will all go so much faster than you think and you'll find yourself ordering high school graduation announcements before you realize.

Made in the USA
Lexington, KY
22 July 2018